Wound Care for Health Professionals

Gerald Bennett

Senior Lecturer
Department of Health Care of the Elderly
The Royal London Hospital (Mile End)
London
UK

and

Marion Moody

Clinical Specialist in Tissue Viability and Wound Care
Institute of Health and Community Services
Bournemouth University
Bournemouth
UK

Jo Campling

Commissioning Editorial Consultant

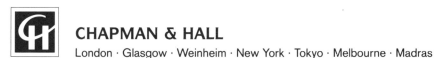

CHAPMAN & HALL
London · Glasgow · Weinheim · New York · Tokyo · Melbourne · Madras

Published by Chapman & Hall, 2–6 Boundary Row, London SE1 8HN, UK

Chapman & Hall, 2–6 Boundary Row, London SE1 8HN, UK

Blackie Academic & Professional, Wester Cleddens Road, Bishopbriggs, Glasgow G64 2NZ, UK

Chapman & Hall GmbH, Pappelallee 3, 69469 Weinheim, Germany

Chapman & Hall USA, 115 Fifth Avenue, New York, NY 10003, USA

Chapman & Hall Japan, ITP-Japan, Kyowa Building, 3F, 2-2-1 Hirakawacho, Chiyoda-ku, Tokyo 102, Japan

Chapman & Hall Australia, 102 Dodds Street, South Melbourne, Victoria 3205, Australia

Chapman & Hall India, R. Seshadri, 32 Second Main Road, CIT East, Madras 600 035, India

Distributed in the USA and Canada by Singular Publishing Group Inc., 4284 41st Street, San Diego, California 92105

First edition 1995

© 1995 Gerald Bennett and Marion Moody

Typeset in Palatino 10/12pt by Mews Photosetting, Beckenham, Kent
Printed in Great Britain by The University Press, Cambridge

ISBN 0 412 55650 2   1 56593 348 6 (USA)

A catalogue record for this book is available from the British Library

Library of Congress Catalog Card Number: 94-74688

∞ Printed on permanent acid-free text paper, manufactured in accordance with ANSI/NISO Z39.48-1992 and ANSI/NISO Z39.48-1984 (Permanence of Paper).

Contents

Acknowledgements

The authors are deeply indebted to Mrs Sam Barnett for her pains-taking work in preparing this manuscript and to patients and colleagues without whose support this manuscript would not have been produced.

We are especially grateful to Mr Peter Thompson for his contribution in Chapter 7 on burns.

Introduction

Wound care is an area of medicine and nursing that is undergoing both a critical evaluation and a clinical renaissance. There are complex reasons for this dual phenomenon. The total cost of providing wound care to the NHS is unknown but serious estimates are in the range of £1 billion – including prevention, management, equipment, dressings, drugs, health care professional time, hospital bed costs, community clinics, education and finally litigation.

It is not surprising, then, that an area of health care that involves practically every specialty and has relevance to all patients, as well as being expensive, should, in the world of cost–benefit analysis, be assessed. Put under scrutiny, wound care in the NHS can be shown to be at best patchy and at worst almost non-existent. There are a few centres of excellence, many of mediocrity and some with standards unworthy of an organization with the calibre of what is still (just about) the most comprehensive free at source sociomedical institution in the world. How has the specialty of wound care arrived at this difficult juncture?

Wounds have obviously been with us since the dawn of humanity. Chronic wounds appear to be no exception with Biblical references, and ancient Egyptian interest as well as the insights of wise medical theologians such as Ambrose Paré. The topic was of interest to all the leading medical experts of their day, such as Fabricius, Brown-Sequard and Paget. It is obvious that chronic wounds taxed the skills of the medical profession but in turn that led to continued interest and observation. The climate changed with the work of the leading physician of his day, Charcot. Based at the huge hospital at Saltpetriere just outside Paris, he became recognized as the most important medical opinion of his generation. In common with other physicians, he and his team began to investigate chronic wounds, pressure sores especially. Charcot was convinced that sustained pressure caused the release of a muscle-destroying 'humour' from damaged nerves. This substance could not be identified and the doctor's interest moved on. The sequelae were profound, however.

If chronic wounds were not an interest for Charcot they were not of interest to the rest of the medical profession. Chronic wounds were moved into the domain of the nurses, a place they have basically retained ever since. Surrounded by medical disinterest the nursing profession has developed wound care into one of its flagship areas, providing research based information on many of its complex factors. The two world wars provided a new impetus for medical interest but this was patchy and involved only a few areas: plastic surgery, physiological measurement and biomechanics. Mainstream medicine kept its distance, encouraged by now by a certain degree of nursing hostility in some places.

It took the pharmaceutical companies to see the potential in this area and nurses were courted to use the latest wound dressings. Wound care (prevention and treatment equipment, dressings, drugs and development areas such as growth factors) is now a multibillion pound industry in the UK alone. Spiralling unevaluated costs are one reason to look more closely at what we do; the other is the contention that there is a better way.

The death of a small amount of heart tissue (heart attack or myocardial infarction) has led to the development of a complex suborganization within the NHS. The heart is an emotive organ and the resulting damage can lead to death, heart failure, arrhythmias, etc. To cope with this we have developed dedicated cardiac units with highly specialized nurses and doctors with an enormous back-up of technical expertise. In addition, vast resources are spent on training; there can scarcely be a medical or nursing student, let alone lay person, who doesn't know what to do when the heart stops suddenly. In addition, attention is now being turned upon prevention involving such issues as exercise, diet and family history.

Contrast this scenario with the death of large areas of tissue on legs, buttocks or hips. This damage is visible, often huge but somewhat unpleasant. It can lead to death or multisystem complications. Its causes are as well known as the cardiac ones yet where are the wound care units in every district general hospital? Where are the specially trained doctors and nurses, the undergraduate curricula for students, the knowledge base that would help patients avoid such distress? By and large they don't exist.

What is needed is a government sponsored comprehensive reorganization of the provision of wound care. There are centres of excellence on which to adopt plans. There are experts in every specialty allied to wounds (general nursing, clinical nurse specialist, general medicine, dermatology, care of the elderly, biomechanics, dietetics, plastic surgery, microbiology, pharmacy, researchers and the industrial conglomerates). The theme is multidisciplinary and seamless (between hospital and community). Care involves a partnership between team member and client to achieve the best result. Care involves education of professionals and specially of potential at-risk groups – the elderly, chronically disabled or immobile. Care involves prevention at all interfaces, be they in hospital or community. Wound care is done badly and inappropriately expensively when ad hoc, using untrained staff in an atmosphere of inadequate knowledge. It is done well in a well trained, motivated multidisciplinary setting, using research tested equipment, dressings, drugs and techniques involving a well informed client.

This book sets out the knowledge base to motivate and hopefully empower the health care worker involved in looking after wounds. The basics of normal skin, the ageing process, wound repair and the assessment of wounds are covered first to give the reader a grounding (or refresher) in the subject. General principles in wound management are then covered, moving on to detailed reviews of the most common chronic wounds – pressure sores and leg ulcers. Other chronic wounds and difficult wounds are covered. No text about wounds would now be complete without advice concerning legal issues plus developments concerning specialist wound care units and the role of education, both professional and for the client.

The field of wound care needs to undergo a revolution. We hope this text helps to speed that process.

Normal skin, subcutaneous and deeper tissues and the process of ageing

1

NORMAL SKIN

It is well known that skin forms our largest organ. To better understand the changes that occur with ageing and as a result of disease it is important to have a working knowledge of the structure and function of skin. There are three distinct layers to normal skin:

1. epidermis
2. dermis
3. skin appendages – sweat glands (apocrine and eccrine)
                        sebaceous glands
                        hair follicles.

Normal skin is shown diagrammatically in Figure 1.1.

THE EPIDERMIS

This is the outer layer of the skin, the thin superficial surface sheet helping the skin perform its many functions, temperature control, protective (physical, chemical, ultraviolet) and sensual. There are four distinct layers which make up the epidermis; from the outside in, these are:

1. the cornified layer (stratum corneum)
2. the granular layer
3. the germinative layer (prickle cell layer)
4. the basal layer.

The main skin cell is the keratinocyte and these undergo cell division in the basal layer and then reside mainly in the germinative layer. By the time these cells reach the granular layer they are losing or have lost their nuclei. The epidermis varies in thickness around the body with the layers being most distinct where the skin is weight bearing, i.e. the sole of the foot.

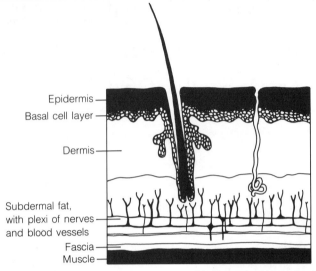

Epidermis
Basal cell layer
Dermis
Subdermal fat, with plexi of nerves and blood vessels
Fascia
Muscle

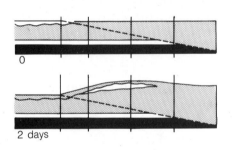

0

2 days

(a) Cross section showing structural features. The bases of the hair follicle and sweat glands reach down into the subdermal fat and are enclosed by basal cells; these are the source of new epithelium when the dermis has been destroyed.

(b) Heat damaged skin giving rise to (1) Superficial, (2) Superficial dermal, (3) Deep dermal and (4) Full thickness burn.

(c) Two days after injury. Increased permeability has caused swelling. Blistering occurs in those tissues which retain a functioning vascular bed and is therefore absent in the deep burn.

Figure 1.1 Normal skin.

There are four cell types seen in the epidermis:

1. keratinocyte – the main cell type
2. melanocyte – the pigment producing cell
3. Langerhans cell – part of the skin's immune system
4. Merkel cell – involved with sensation and chemical production.

Keratinocytes

These are the main epidermal cells and cell division takes place in the basal layer with one of the new cells formed migrating upwards towards the surface. As it does so the nucleus disappears and the cell dies, forming the surface stratum corneum. Keratinocytes are connected to each other in the prickle cell layer by filaments or desmosomes and in the basal layer are connected by hemidesmosomes to the underlying basement membrane. These connections become important in various disease processes; for example, the basal layer separates from the basement membrane in the blistering disease epidermolysis bullosa. Other disease processes such as dermatitis make the desmosomes swollen and oedematous but their role in pressure damage or venous or arterial leg ulceration is not known. As the keratinocyte cells enter and subsequently leave the granular layer they are said to mature, a process called orthokeratosis. In some areas of the body the skin surface must remain moist, e.g. inside the mouth. In these situations the epidermis is different and instead of a granular layer there is an outer layer of nucleated squamous cells. This process is called physiological parakeratosis which can occur in other situations. If keratinocytes are grown artificially in cell culture they will not form a stratum corneum (parakeratosis, not orthokeratosis). In the disease psoriasis, something goes wrong with the formation of a normal stratum corneum and a faster imperfect outer layer is formed (pathological parakeratosis). It is estimated to take a keratinocyte four weeks to go from basal layer to stratum corneum (four days in psoriasis).

Desmosomes are not the only binding link between keratinocytes. The cells also produce a protein – alpha-keratin – which forms filaments (tonofilaments) running into the desmosomes. These links help provide surface strength and the cells also produce fatty substances (epidermal lipids) to supplement the waterproofing and suppleness needed. Recently it has been shown that the epidermal keratinocytes also play a role in the skin's immunosurveillance system by producing immunologically active substances.

Melanocytes

Epidermal melanocytes produce the pigment melanin. The number of melanocytes varies around the body (more in light exposed areas) but not between black and white races (black races produce more melanin). Melanin is produced by a chemical reaction (involving the enzymes dopaoxidase and tyrosinase) and passes along connecting processes (dendrites) to the surrounding keratinocytes (the so-called epidermal melanin unit). The pigment is protective for ultraviolet light and melanocytes occur predominantly in the epidermis, eye and hair bulb. This protective process appears generally good in that malignant tumours of this cell type are comparatively rare in black races. The same is not true in white, sun exposed populations where malignant melanoma, a potentially fatal disorder, is reaching record levels [1,2]. The analogy with the 'ageing' effects of UV light on skin is interesting. The last few decades have seen the social image of sunbathing as healthy and desirable, even sexy. This contrasts with the Victorian era when pale was considered beautiful. The message is beginning to get across that UV exposures, especially in childhood, is not at all healthy yet the pharmaceutical response has geared itself more to the antiageing aspects (blocking UVA) rather than the very unsexy blocking of cancer. Malignant melanoma appears to be yet another preventable condition and current knowledge indicates that only two exposures to intense UV light (sunburn) in childhood put you in a high risk category for developing malignant melanoma as an adult. The situation is such that in Australia dermatology teams visit the beaches to advise on sun exposure and pigmented skin lesions.

Langerhans cells

Though discovered in 1860 by Paul Langerhans when he was still a medical student, it is only comparatively recently that the immuno-logical nature of the cell has been realized. It is derived from the bone marrow and is in contact with fellow Langerhans cells by means of connections (dendrites). It is thought that its role in the epider-mis is to come into contact first with the numerous antigens presented to the body; hence it will probably prove to have a crucial role in the allergic/immunological skin disorders such as contact dermatitis and inflammatory reactions.

The basement membrane

This structure divides the epidermis from the next distinct layer, the dermis. It appears to be a flexible and permeable membrane uniting the two layers on either side. Diseases of this layer illustrate how it works because in both the genetically based epidermolysis bullosa and the autoimmune condition of bullous pemphigoid, the epidermis and dermis separate leaving a raw dermal surface.

THE DERMIS

The dermis is mainly made up of type 1 collagen (a supporting or struc-tural framework of protein fibres) held together by bridges or bonds. Interspersed within this framework are elastin (elastic) fibres adding suppleness and improved tensile strength. This structure is within a fibrous complex substance called dermal proteoglycans. It is thus a fibrous, tough and elastic layer well supplied with blood vessels, nerves and lymphatics as well as three types of cell:

1. fibroblast – produces collagen
2. macrophage – hunter cell, especially important in infection
3. mast cell – part of the skin's immune system.

The dermis and epidermis are supplied with blood via a complex network of vessels. They form superficial and deep layers with a communicating system. This vasculature is capable of responding to numerous insults and copes with low temperatures, volume loss and anxiety or fear with intense vasoconstriction (shutting down of the skin blood supply). In contrast, high temperatures, exercise and some skin diseases (erythroderma) cause vasodilatation, redness and sweating. Microscopic dermal lymphatic channels run into the local lymph node chain. The dermis is the site for the nerve endings concerned with touch, heat and cold perception and proprioception (the position of a digit or limb in space). These free nerve endings are not evenly distributed, with certain areas more sensitive to different stimuli, e.g. finger tips, genital area, tongue, lips, etc. There are also some specialized receptors present in the dermis, e.g. the Pacinian corpuscle which allows for the sensation of deep pressure and the Meissner corpuscle (involved in the nerve endings around the base of hairs).

SKIN APPENDAGES

These consist of:

- hair follicle
- sebaceous gland
- arrector pili muscle
- eccrine sweat glands
- apocrine glands (axilla)
- nails (modified skin appendage).

The hair follicle is made up of a hair shaft and its hair bulb papilla. The shaft is layered with an outer cortex and inner medulla, while the bulb has a good blood supply. Three different types of hair are recognized: the terminal hair of the scalp, the terminal hair (hormone dependent) of the male chin, axilla and pubic area and the fine downy vellous hair seen on many body sites.

The scalp hair cycle is complex but established. There are three phases – anagen (growing), catagen (resting) and telogen (shedding). These phases are randomly distributed across the scalp and at any one time 80% of hair growth is in the anagen phase with the remainder in either catagen or telogen. Sebaceous glands occur at the base of hair follicles and their secretion sebum travels via the hair follicle to the surface. The size and production of the glands is hormone dependent and in an overactive state they produce conditions such as acne, especially where there is a high proportion of sebaceous glands, such as on the face, back and chest. Eccrine sweat glands occur all over the body whereas apocrine sweat glands are found mainly in the axilla and the groin.

The arrector pili muscles are attached to both hair follicle and dermis. Upon contraction the hair follicle is pulled into a more perpendicular position and the nearby sebaceous gland is squeezed. At the same time the dermis is pulled downwards causing a small depression, the so-called goose pimples or goose flesh.

Nails consist of a nail plate which rests on a vascular nail bed. The nail proper grows outwards protected by a skin covering, the cuticle. The base of the nail, the lunula, is paler and usually semicircular. Damage to the nail plate is thought to account for ridges that often occur and systemic diseases can cause nail colour changes as well as banding or horizontal nail colour changes. Hard, horny nails can be seen in elderly people (onychogryphosis) (Figure 1.2) and nail plate trauma is one theory.

SUBCUTANEOUS AND DEEPER TISSUES

Beneath the dermis lies the subcutaneous fat. The depth of this layer varies according to body site (small amounts usually on arms, legs,

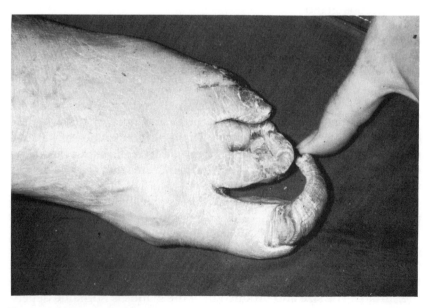

Figure 1.2 Onychogryphosis.

back and large amounts over buttocks) and disposition, e.g. obese or not. This layer provides a pressure cushioning effect and is also important in temperature regulation. Subcutaneous fat has a comparatively poor blood supply and hence tends to heal slowly following damage.

Underlying this fatty layer are the deeper tissues – muscles, tendons, joint capsules and finally bones. These deeper structures tend to have a much better blood, nerve and lymphatic supply. They assume crucial importance when the integrity of the epidermis and dermis is compromised either by a deep wound or via pressure. The damage caused by pressure can be proportionately worse the deeper the site, with the highest interface pressures deep down where a bony prominence abuts against muscle (Figure 1.3).

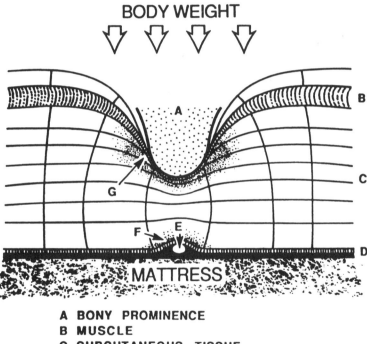

A BONY PROMINENCE
B MUSCLE
C SUBCUTANEOUS TISSUE
D SKIN
E CATHETER SPIGOT
F SUPERFICIAL PRESSURE NECROSIS
G DEEP PRESSURE NECROSIS

Figure 1.3 Pressure sore - possible aetiological model. Reproduced with permission from Bliss, M.R. (1992) Pressure sore management and prevention, in *Textbook of Geriatric Medicine and Gerontology*, 4th edn, (eds J.C. Brocklehurst, R.C. Tallis and H.M. Fillet), Churchill Livingstone, Edinburgh, p. 923.

SKIN AND THE AGEING PROCESS

> We are ignorant of the basic scientific processes underlying wound healing . . . this ignorance and our resulting deficiencies in clinical management means that the majority of wounds are being maintained by nursing and medical care, not cured. [3]

This ignorance of the basic scientific facts about healing has until recently been mirrored by our ignorance of the issues surrounding the ageing process. Gerontology, the scientific study of ageing, has been and remains a Cinderella specialty tainted with the image of quackery and elixirs of youth. The famous neurologist Brown-Sequard was shunned by his medical colleagues when he developed a rejuvenating serum and published before and after photographs. The concept of a rejuvenating serum composed of guinea-pig and chimpanzee testes was ridiculed. Similar sentiments surrounded the published works arising from the then Eastern bloc countries Romania, Poland and East Germany reporting longevity experiments with rats. It took similar studies in the UK and USA before there was confirmation of increased lifespan by modifying the diet of rats (reducing the calorie intake before puberty) and the use of antioxidants to mop up what are seen as harmful free radical particles within cells. Dame Barbara Cartland has long espoused the value of vitamin E (amongst other things) to not so faint ridicule until vitamin E was discovered to be one of the most potent antioxidants and now half the population appear to be taking it.

As we age we become more prone to an increasing number of disease processes (pathology). The mistake was made, however, of confusing these disease processes with normal ageing (physiology). So fundamental has this mistake been that it is still not understood by the majority of health care professionals, even those dealing with elderly people. Professor Bernard Isaacs coined the term 'geriatric giants' to illustrate the point [4]. He listed the medical ways in which many frail elderly people present with a disease process:

- falls
- confusion
- incontinence
- immobility

to which has been added

- pressure sores.

These are symptoms of disease, which can be as diverse as a urinary tract infection, myocardial infarction (heart attack) or kidney or heart failure. The same analogy can be made with children. A fit or seizure in a child is not epilepsy. The fit is a symptom of illness which could be meningitis, brain tumour, febrile illness, trauma or epilepsy.

It therefore follows that it is not normal ageing for an elderly person to be confused, fall about or be incontinent, yet the majority of the population accept these as facts about growing old, as do elderly people themselves, and hence do not seek help. The concept of normal ageing can be made clearer by reference to the work of an American gerontologist, Strehler [5]. He set out a framework by which all processes could be evaluated to decide if they were normal ageing (physiology) or not, i.e. disease (pathology):

- Universal
- Intrinsic
- Irreversible
- Deleterious.

His proposal is that one can think of any process and apply these principles. If it obeys all four then it is a true ageing process, if not then it is a disease process. An example is hypertension (high blood pressure). This falls at the first hurdle because although extremely common in Western affluent communities secondary to atheroma (hardening of the arteries), there are many populations around the world where blood pressure remains stable with increasing age and hence it is not universal. On the other hand, cataract formation is probably a true ageing process. Clear vision is maintained by the lens of the eye adapting its shape as the surrounding muscles either contract or relax. New lens fibres, however, form around the lens like numerous skins around an onion. No layers are lost but they continue to pack down making the lens firmer and less easily moulded as the muscles relax and contract. Finally the lens cannot alter shape at all and the numerous outer layers begin to make the lens opaque (cataract) until the dull white opacity is clearly visible. Even in elderly people with good vision this process can be found with careful examination of the eye and the process obeys all of Strehler's four criteria.

Using these gerontological principles means that we have to rethink most of what has become standard information concerning skin and ageing. The knowledge base has to be rewritten. This can best be illustrated by referral to Figures 1.4 and 1.5. These photographs show some of the skin changes that have erroneously been attributed to the ageing process:

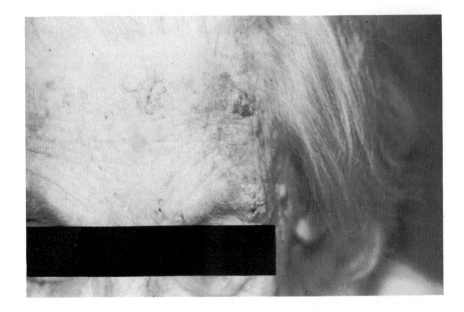

Figure 1.4 Effects of ultraviolet light on face.

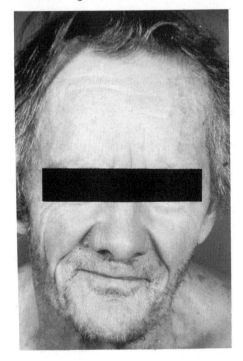

Figure 1.5 Effects of ultraviolet light on face.

- wrinkles
- pigmentation
- depigmentation
- telangiectasia
- benign and malignant skin tumours
- thin/transparent skin.

Other 'ageing' skin processes have included dryness, itchiness (senile pruritus) and bruising (senile purpura). It is now apparent that most of the above changes are due to the skin's exposure to ultraviolet light, the so-called photoageing of UVA. This is why the changes are most pronounced over those areas habitually exposed to sunlight, the face, hands and arms. There is a genetic component to wrinkles (relatives of W.H. Auden may find them hard to avoid completely) but the main determinant is sun. Ultraviolet light affects both epidermis and dermis, acting on the collagen substrate and causing thin skin. In some severely affected individuals the skin becomes akin to tissue paper with purpura and skin tears occurring without trauma. This is the so-called transparent skin syndrome (Figure 1.6). The weakened and thinned collagen fails to support the blood vessels in the dermis and hence they break easily. The blood breakdown mechanism is also affected so that the bruises do not change colour quickly and remain visible for many months.

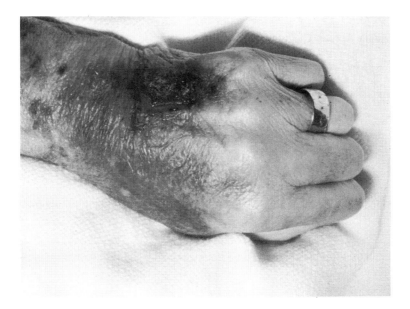

Figure 1.6 Transparent skin syndrome.

Normal skin ageing is, therefore, quite a benign affair. The epidermis becomes slightly thinner and the dermis changes with some reduction in the amounts of extracellular matrix proteins, collagen and elastin. These changes are still most marked, however, in the sun exposed areas. Predominantly covered skin, i.e. the abdomen, 'ages' very little and one would be hard pressed to determine someone's age if only their abdomen were uncovered. There also appears to be a slight reduction in transcutaneous oxygen consumption when measured in elderly people though the majority of scientific work on elderly skin has not been performed using health status defined populations, i.e. normal fit elderly people. Only in this way will the true ageing processes be demonstrated and not the effects of disease on the organ that tends to mirror internal disorders best.

The effect of ageing on the wound healing/repair mechanisms such as keratinocytes and growth factors will be described in the following chapter on wound repair.

REFERENCES

1. MacKie, R.M. Smyth, J.F., Soutar, D.S. *et al*. (1985) Malignant melanoma in Scotland 1979–1983. *Lancet*, **ii**, 859–62.
2. MacKie, R.M. (1983) Malignant melanoma. Pigment cell, in *Epidemiology of Malignant Melanoma: 10 Years Progress*, (ed. R.M. MacKie), S. Karger, Basel, pp. 1–21.
3. Ferguson, M. (1993) Paper presented at the Wound Healing and Ageing Workshop, King's Fund, London, 2 March.
4. Isaacs, B. (1976) *The Giants of Geriatrics: A Study of Symptoms of Old Age*. Inaugural lecture, University of Birmingham.
5. Strehler, B.L. (ed.) (1964, 1967) *Advances in Gerontological Research*, Vols 1 & 2, Academic Press, New York.

Wound healing

2

Any damage to skin integrity, from minor abrasions to major tissue loss, results in a complex process of wound healing. This may mean the formation of scar tissue. There are many factors that can affect wound healing including oxygen, nutrition (especially Vitamin C, zinc), steroids and the type of dressing used. The process of ageing and wound healing deserves special consideration. Failure of wound repair mechanisms can also have many causes, the most common and important being infection.

The initial injury to the superficial and deeper layers of the skin initiates the wound healing response, a sort of cascade mechanism that involves specific key cells. The response is ordered with some predetermined time limits though these can be adversely affected by many things including infection. The role of a good oxygen supply is crucial, as is the overall general health of the individual; wound healing cannot be considered in isolation from the whole person. Key components include:

- capillaries
- neutrophils
- monocytes/macrophages
- fibroblasts
- collagen
- oxygen
- growth factors.

The process of wound repair (mainly uncomplicated surgical wounds) has been extensively studied. The timings and sequencing appear to be as follows.

As soon as injury occurs the protective mechanism of blood clotting tries to fill the space and unite the sides of the injury. The fibrin (blood protein) clot thus includes red blood cells, any dead tissue and any foreign tissue that may have entered the wound. The surface part of this usually dries out. Inside at a histological level white blood cells (neutrophils) appear after about eight hours followed by monocytes (precursors to macrophages) after about 24 hours.

Neutrophils try and combat any infection present (by attacking bacteria) and monocytes help as scavenger cells. As more macrophages appear these in turn stimulate fibroblasts, the cells that produce collagen and help induce new capillaries to grow into the wound. In addition lymphocytes (white cells important in the immune system) also appear and the collection and activity of these cells is responsible for the process known as inflammation. This is a normal part of the wound healing process and in itself does not signify wound infection. Inflammation involves some redness (erythema) around the wound and a slight increase in temperature (both locally and, in large wounds, systemically).

The blood cells appear to be attracted and directed to the wound by a series of complex messages including substances called growth factors (expanded upon later). The blood cells are also dependent on other things, one of the most important being oxygen. Macrophages appear to need less oxygen so can survive further away from the underlying capillary supply. They tend to occur at the edges of the wound [1]. Fibroblasts, however, appear to be critically dependent on an adequate oxygen supply and hence are found much closer to the capillary bed and indeed fibroblasts and capillaries develop together as a unit [2].

INFLAMMATION

The process known as inflammation is proving to be a highly complex interaction of biochemical and cellular actions. The knowledge base is now enormous but a brief expansion upon the facts already given will hopefully explain and stimulate further reading. Each part of the inflammatory process has both stimulatory and regulatory or inhibitory systems to control it. Substances known as mediators can have local or general effects or in turn induce other cells to release different mediators. These substances can attract, repel or activate cells used in the inflammatory process.

The process of inflammation is a sequential one allowing the body to protect itself from further damage. This takes the form of killing bacteria, etc., dealing with toxins and foreign bodies and trying to wall off damaged tissue. The epidermis is the first layer of skin to respond to inflammation. It does so in a variety of ways including hyperproliferation of keratinocytes with the release of keratinocyte enzymes. These include acid phosphatase, used in nucleic acid degradation, and induced by ultraviolet light exposure and the application of vitamin A. Other enzymes include acidic protease cathepsins which appear to act by chemotaxis and attract neutrophils, thus continuing the inflammatory response.

LEUCOCYTES

Neutrophils are the most common of the leucocytes (white blood cells). They mature from stem cells in the bone marrow, circulate and then enter tissues. In inflammation and especially when this is due to infection, huge numbers are produced, eventually depleting all the mature forms so that less mature cells appear in the blood. The cytoplasm of the neutrophil contains granules filled with enzymes. Neutrophils work by ingesting the foreign material (phagocytosis) and destroying it enzymatically. Many cells die in the process, releasing their enzymes and other contents and in severe cases pus is formed. Neutrophils also release a stored pyrogen (a substance that raises the body temperature) contributing to the fever often seen in inflammatory conditions. Many of the substances released have chemotactic properties (they attract other types of cell to the site of injury).

Eosinophils are a type of neutrophil (mobile and phagocytic) but only found in large numbers in specific conditions such as asthma, parasitic infestations, burns and lymphomas. They appear to be under the control of substances released by T-lymphocytes.

Mast cells and basophils are leucocytes involved in acute inflammatory conditions such as urticaria and angio-oedema. Mast cells come from two sources: mucosal type mast cells (dependent on T-lymphocytes for maturation) and connective tissue mast cells (which mainly occur in skin and release histamine). Basophils are leucocytes with less enzymatic activity in their cytoplasm. They only occur in small numbers and are found in delayed hypersensitivity reactions.

MONOCTYES AND MACROPHAGES
(THE MONONUCLEAR PHAGOCYTE SYSTEM)

Monocytes mature in the bone marrow and then, like neutrophils, they enter the circulation and finally the tissues. Some stay within a tissue and are called histiocytes. They still form part of the mononuclear phagocyte system (previously known as the reticulo-endothelial system). The others continue to mature and eventually become macrophages (with the ability to be phagocytic and secrete substances). In inflammation large numbers are formed and others mobilized from various parts of the body. Macrophages are highly complex and do a variety of things. They seek and phagocytose micro-organisms. They store debris and stimulate lymphoid cells to produce antibodies. They release a large number of stored enzymes which help prolong the inflammatory response and break down tissues. It is now known that some of the substances released feed back to the macrophage, allowing it to monitor the response and if necessary release more. In certain circumstances macrophages can develop into giant cells. This appears to be a way of a cell storing a material it can't otherwise deal with (by destroying or excreting). These cells are found in granulomas, often within chronic lesions.

MEDIATORS OF INFLAMMATION

A large number of pharmacologically active substances are involved in the inflammatory process and come from the leucocytes, the damaged tissue and plasma. Some interact and indeed stimulate other pathways, enhancing an effect. If a substance affects the immunological activity of a cell it is called a cytokine. Some of the different mediators are mentioned briefly below.

Histamine is made and stored in the granules of mast cells. On its release there are at least two different receptor types: H1 and H2. H1 is involved in blood vessel changes (increased permeability and dilatation) as well as smooth muscle contraction. H2 increases gastric acid production by stimulating gastric parietal cell secretion.

Enzymatic activity on cell membranes releases fatty acids. One, arachidonic acid, is very important during inflammation. It is the precursor of prostaglandins (with active effects on the blood vessels of the skin and smooth muscle, especially in the lungs) and leukotrienes (again affecting smooth muscle, blood vessels and mucus production) as well as prostacyclin (a potent inhibitor of platelet aggregation).

Interleukins are cytokines involved in both inflammation and wound healing. They are formed as a result of skin damage and appear to influence T and B-lymphocyte activity, epithelial, endothelial and fibroblast cell activity and activate leucocytes.

Interferon derived from various sources (macrophages, fibroblasts and lymphocytes) is also involved in the inflammatory process. The different interferons affect the immune process and other cytokines.

Neuropeptides (e.g. somatostatin and substance P) are part of the mast cell/histamine response and involved in the associated weal and flare. During the process of inflammation plasma proteins (known as acute phase proteins) develop anti-inflammatory properties. One, C-reactive protein, is produced within the first 48 hours of an infection. It activates the complement cascade (with many parts of the complement series having anti-inflammatory properties) as well as stimulating leucocytosis and encouraging phagocytosis.

Lysosomes are the membrane bound packets of enzymes found within a cell's cytoplasm. They form part of the phagocytic function of the cell as well as being involved in the inflammatory response when released extracellularly. The specific enzymes within each lysosome are determined by the cell type but include acid phosphatase, proteases and hydrolases [3].

Fibroblasts make substances called glycosaminoglycans (the bricks) and fibronectin (the cement) which together form collagen. Fibroblasts also produce other forms of connective tissue. The collagen formed in the wound situation, however, is very different from the collagen produced in normal skin. The collagen of normal skin is set out in an organized framework of large bundles, each large fibre made up of smaller ones linked by crossbands. Wound collagen fails to organize itself well, with large fibres irregularly arranged and without all the crosslinks. Five types of collagen are recognized [2].

- type 1 – mature skin, tendon and bone
- type 2 – cartilage
- type 3 – cardiovascular tissues, infant skin and the granulation tissue of healing skin wounds
- type 4 – basement membranes
- type 5 – basement membranes.

The fact that the new wound collagen is less organized also means that it is less strong and these mechanical aspects of wound healing have been summarized by Forrester [2]. He describes three distinct phases in the repair process:

1. The phase of preparation – marked enzyme and cellular activity but no recordable tensile strength in the wound.
2. The phase of proliferation – the fibroblast-capillary system is most active (from 4–5 days after the wound) and tensile strength rises rapidly as collagen is formed.
3. The phase of maturation – after a month or so strength recovers more slowly and the cellular and vascular activity reduces progressively. After five months scar tissue still only has half the ability of normal tissues to resist rupture. There is good evidence, however, that growth factors can not only improve general healing but when applied shortly after the trauma, specifically increase the tensile strength of newly formed wounds [4,5].

These phases or stages of wound healing merge and many aspects are occurring simultaneously. The stages each have their own biological objectives. In the inflammatory/preparation stage it is obviously damage limitation. The proliferative phase enables replacement of lost tissue volume and encourages the two most important aspects – granulation tissue (from the newly budding and developing capillary system) and epithelialization (the encouragement of migratory epithelial cells from the margins of the wound). The remodelling/maturing stage tries to restore some or all of the structural and functional integrity of the wound. The role here of the newly formed collagen has been mentioned but in open wounds the role of wound contraction in closing wounds is of vital importance. This appears to involve the full thickness of skin and subcutaneous tissues and is initiated by special cells (myofibrils) in the wound margin [6].

SPECIAL FACTORS IN WOUND HEALING

OXYGEN

As one might expect, successful wound healing is dependent upon good oxygen resources. In the early stages of wound healing tissue oxygen is extremely low (<10 mmHg) indicating the absence of a working microcirculation [7]. The important cells – fibroblasts, neutrophils and macrophages – can survive in this environment but cannot carry out their special functions. Thus collagen is not produced or micro-organisms killed. In this low oxygen environment, however, the macrophages promote new capillary formation (angiogenic role) thus helping to improve the circulation and raise the tissue oxygen [8]. Once the tissue oxygen improves (>10 mmHg means that collagen can be synthesized) the wound healing process can continue apace. Tissue oxygenation has both local and more distant factors. The local ones include the vascularity of the tissue (the more vascular the area, the faster the wound healing) as well as the blood flow to that area. The more distant rate limiting features include cardiac or pulmonary disease (which can obviously cause general hypoxic states) and general or local vasoconstriction limiting blood flow. Haematological conditions such as hyperviscosity (thickened and slow moving blood) may also alter tissue oxygenation, as may anaemia.

There is evidence that when oxygen delivery is poor to an already ischaemic area the blood vessel reacts by first suffering endothelial lining damage. This makes the capillary leak fluid, forming oedema which in turn makes the oxygen situation worse. One therapeutic measure undergoing evaluation is the use of hyperbaric oxygen (HBO) therapy [9]. This is the administration of elevated partial pressures of oxygen to try and restore normal oxygen levels in hypoxic areas. The current most common use of this form of therapy is in the treatment of arterial leg ulcers, i.e. more oxygen delivered in the same diminished amount of blood reaching the site. There are whole body chambers where a person is enclosed in a pressurized environment filled with air and breathes 100% oxygen. This forces more oxygen into solution in the plasma (oxygen is carried both attached with haemoglobin and dissolved in plasma) and hopefully supplies ischaemic tissue with enough oxygen to heal. Whole body chambers are obviously expensive and the situation may become complex to manage. Trials are taking place with local hyperbaric oxygen cylinders into which the affected limb is placed and the chamber then acts as a mini HBO system.

GROWTH FACTORS

Growth factors are peptides (proteins) that have an influence over cell proliferation and hence are vital in wound healing. They are a complex phenomenon attracting enormous amounts of time and resources from basic scientists to pharmaceutical companies. The knowledge base is expanding rapidly and changing almost daily. Growth factors have been named after the target cell or source that led to their discovery. However, it is now known that individual growth factors affect more than one type of cell and probably work with other growth factors though the timings and relative concentrations needed for maximal effects are still unclear. In addition they may not always be 'growth' factors for in some situations they are known to inhibit cell proliferation.

Their action has been likened to a form of language controlling wound healing. Each growth factor forms a 'letter' of the alphabet in the overall language concept, with other factors (the state or activation of the wound) also important in organizing the 'words' [10].

Growth factors can be differentiated thus:

- paracrine – act upon the neighbouring cell
- autocrine – act upon the producing cell
- three types – 1. signal proliferation
               2. stimulate migration
               3. alter phenotypic state.

The major growth factors have been described and listed by Glover [11]. The list includes:

- epidermal growth factor (EGF)
- platelet derived growth factor (PDGF)
- transforming growth factors alpha and beta (TGF-α and TGF-β)
- interleukin-1 (IL-1)
- tumour necrosis factor alpha (TNF-α)
- fibroblast growth factor (FGF).

EGF derives its name from the fact that its first known action was on epidermal basal cell proliferation. It has been found in body fluids and its receptor sites are present on all cell membranes apart from the blood forming (haematopoietic) system. Its known actions now include increased proliferation of keratinocytes, corneal epithelium, mammary gland epithelium, endothelial cells and fibroblasts. It also causes an increased synthesis of the connective tissue glycosaminoglycans (part of the collagen system) by human fibroblasts. It is thus vital in the wound repair/healing mechanism.

PDGF is stored in the α-granules of platelets and is thus released during the clotting process immediately after tissue damage. It is a potent vasoconstrictor (important in the early stages of wound haemostatic control) and it encourages the general activity around fibroblasts. It also pulls in chemotactically fibroblasts, smooth muscle cells, monocytes and neutrophils and thus helps develop granulation tissue, one of the most vital components of wound healing.

TGF-α is very similar to EGF and it is described as the major factor in normal keratinocyte (major skin cell type) replication. It also promotes new vessel formation. TGF-β has both stimulatory and inhibitory capabilities. It inhibits the growth of keratinocytes, hepatocytes, T and B-lymphocytes and bronchial epithelial cells. It stimulates the proliferation of fibroblasts and osteoblasts as well as promoting the formation of glycosaminoglycans and collagen. It is a potent immunosuppressive agent.

IL-1 is part of the human defence system released by cells after injury (e.g. neutrophils, monocytes and keratinocytes). It stimulates the proliferation of many of the basic wound healing cells.

TNF-α appears to have many effects including activating neutrophils, macrophages and lymphocytes. It was originally discovered as being responsible for the haemorrhagic necrosis of tumours in animals.

FGF promotes cartilage repair and alters the amount of the various types of collagen made by cells.

From Glover's analysis [11] it is easy to see why growth factors are eliciting so much interest. However, the main studies have been carried out on animal models which does not form a good basis from which to extract information concerning human wounds, especially the chronic forms in leg ulcers and pressure sores. In addition there are many questions concerning growth factors that have yet to be answered. What is the interaction between the growth factors and the extracellular matrix? Does it stabilize the growth factor, protect it from degradation or simply store it long-term? Can the activity of the various growth factors be increased by altering (adding substances to) the extracellular matrix? In addition we are unsure as to the sequencing of growth factor events, their mutual interactions (and in what concentrations) and how they may be used for practical effect (e.g. topically onto the wound, impregnated into the dressing or formed naturally and locally by enhancement or stimulatory techniques).

The individual growth factors have become the property of different pharmaceutical companies and biological agencies. This makes research difficult, especially in the investigation of the actions of the different factors at different times in the wound healing process. There are the research and ethical issues of the use of growth factors from one patient source being used to stimulate wound healing in another, especially while the cost of recombinant factors (bioengineered) precludes their routine use. If these issues can be overcome growth factors may well fulfil the potential scientists have earmarked for them.

NUTRITION

The role of nutrition is now assuming critical importance in the holistic approach to wound healing. A significant proportion of the healing process is local and hence occurs despite nutritional inadequacies, yet in a deficient situation wound healing is either delayed or inadequate. Researchers are now turning their attention to the complex nutritional issues that are involved in the wound repair process [12]. As in so many aspects of wound care, prevention is better than cure. A healthy nutritious diet helps towards good skin integrity, especially in the healing process if that integrity is breached. Nutrition is now considered so important that in elective cases where nutrition is deficient, full assessment followed by many weeks of replacement therapy are now instituted, if possible. Attention is also focusing upon those patients in hospital or in the community who have some form of wound and in addition are deemed either malnourished or suboptimally nourished. The role of nutritional intervention to improve wound healing has necessitated the formation of nutrition teams to advise and if necessary administer appropriate therapy. All clients should have access to this expertise, not only hospital patients.

In order to understand the requirements in a deficient state it is necessary to have a brief overview of the assessment process concerning nutrition and what constitutes the optimal nutritional requirements in normal wound healing. A practical approach to some of the more common deficiency states can then be applied.

Assessment

Body mass/weight usually decreases with age though this is inconclusive and does not cover the very old [13]. One critical factor for

Table 2.1 Effects of trace elements

Trace element	Effects of deficiency relevant to healing	Common causes of deficiency	Repletion/Treatment
Zinc	• Synthesis of all components for tissue repair • Repair of sepsis? • Lymphopenia	• Low intake • Excessive losses • Renal failure, antimetabolite chemotherapy • Impaired zinc? metabolism in some individuals with leg ulcers	• Prevent deficiency in patients at risk; ensure nutritional support contains trace element supplement (e.g. add iodine trace, Kabivitrum in TPN) • Monitor status in high risk patients • Oral zinc supplement effective in healing leg ulcers where serum zinc low • Topical zinc oxide favourably influences healing
Copper	• Collagen synthesis • Anaemia reduces oxygen • Neutropenia, leucopenia	• Excessive losses • Intake in patients on TPN	• Prevent deficiency in patients at risk (see above) • Monitor status in high risk patients
Iron	• Macrocytic anaemia oxygen delivery • Collagen synthesis • Wound tensile strength	• Dietary deficiency • Chronic blood loss	• Dietary supplements • Treat underlying cause • Iron-dextran therapy inappropriate in hypoferraemia of severe injury, stress, sepsis

Reproduced by kind permission of S.G. McLaren and *Wound Management Journal*.

Table 2.2 Effects of vitamins

Vitamins	Effects of deficiency relevant to healing	Common causes of deficiency	Repletion/treatment
C	• Wound tensile strength • Dehiscence • Tissue damage by free radicals (e.g. ischaemia-reperfusion injury) • Capillary fragility • Bleeding • Healing of pressure sores • Risk of sepsis	• Dietary intake • Utilization in injury, sepsis stress	• Supplements in stress, sepsis, severe injury prevent deficiency • Ensure dietary intake/ nutritional support regimen contains vitamin supplements (e.g. Multibionta (Merck); Soliviton N (Kabivitrum) in TPN • Supplements in pressure sores enhance healing – some uncontrolled studies • Effects of megadose supplements controversial • Some studies demonstrate improved immune function with supplements
B complex	• Synthesis of components for tissue repair • Collagen linkage • Tensile strength of wound • Immune response • Risk of sepsis • Macrocytic anaemia O_2 delivery to wound	• Dietary intake • Absorption of folate by sulphonamides, phenytoin • Malabsorption syndromes	• Ensure intake adequate • Supplements in depletion states • Pantothenic acid supplements? Healing of aponeuroses
A	• Collagen crosslinkage • Wound tensile strength • Impaired granulation • Impaired immune defence • Risk sepsis	• Dietary intake • Utilization in severe thermal injury	• Ensure intake adequate • Supplements necessary in burns: caution – over-repletion risks toxicity • Topical application enhances epithelialization in wound with retarded healing
E	• Tissue damage due to free radical formation	• Dietary intake	• Effects of supplements under investigation in healing of venous ulcers

Reproduced by kind permission of S.G. McLaren and *Wound Management Journal.*

nutrition is the energy intake of an individual (if more energy is expended than accumulated, the person will lose weight).The three components of weight that can be studied are body fat mass (fat/adipose tissue), lean body mass (mainly muscle) and skeletal mass (bones). All seem to alter as we get older. Skeletal mass appears to decline (as does bone density), with women more markedly affected. Lean body mass goes down while body fat mass goes up and these changes have been put down to elderly people being less physically active. Practical assessment procedures include [14]:

- measuring body weight accurately and comparing to the 'ideal' age/sex body weight;
- skinfold measurements (using calipers at various body sites, e.g. triceps skinfold);
- measuring body weight sequentially;
- bone densitometry;
- energy expenditure estimated as a proportion of the maximal exercise capacity;
- food intake analysis;
- serum biochemistry interpretation;
- macronutrient estimation/measurement;
- micronutrient estimation/measurement;
- role of disease/drugs.

Basic assessments should be carried out at the earliest opportunity by any member of the multidisciplinary team whereas the more complex assessments and requirement schedules should be the province of the dietitian or nutrition team member.

Essential nutrients in normal wound healing

These can be divided into the macro and micronutrients. Macronutrients include protein/amino acids, fat/fatty acids, glucose and calcium. Micronutrients include zinc, iron, copper and the range of vitamins (Tables 2.1 and 2.2).

Macronutrients

Protein/amino acids

Physical activity appears to be the key point in maintaining lean body mass (mainly muscle but activity probably enhances skeletal mass as well) in older people. It is not known how the decline in lean body mass affects normal protein metabolism but pure protein deficiency is rare with multiple deficiencies being more common. Proteins are obviously essential in normal wound healing and contribute at every stage including proteoglycan and collagen synthesis as well as neoangiogenesis (the formation of the new capillary networks). Marked deficiencies would obviously be expected to delay this process. Serum proteins are an established means of assessing body protein stores. Albumin is the most documented and a low value (less than 35 gm/l) indicates the need for a thorough assessment. As the serum albumin falls there is a correlation with a poor clinical state with eventual oedema formation, poor wound healing and increased complications such as infections. It forms one of the vital baseline tests and is an ongoing measure of nutritional status.

Some amino acids have specific roles to play in wound healing. Generally they form the building blocks for the various cell structures but two, arginine and glutamine, appear to have specific wound healing functions. Arginine enhances collagen synthesis and glutamine stimulates macrophages, lymphocytes and fibroblasts.

Fat/fatty acids

The role of adipose tissue in wound healing remains unclear.There may be a physical action (as seen in delayed wound healing in the obese) and in certain circumstances fat can be used as an energy source. Adipose tissue does have a role in thermoregulation but the connection between this and wound healing is unexplored. Fatty acids are now attracting research interest because of their importance in membrane structure and function. Research is being carried out into polyunsaturated fatty acids (PUFA) and their effects on macrophage function, inflammation and wound healing.

Glucose

This is one of the essential nutrient factors in wound healing, with leucocytes and macrophages needing it as part of the inflammatory process and fibroblasts utilizing it in the formation of collagen.

Calcium

The role of calcium in the skeletal well-being of older people is well established but its role in wound healing is less clear. It is an essential component of most cellular activity but whether this is affected when the body is deficient (i.e. in osteoporosis or in osteomalacia where there is a lack of Vitamin D to ensure absorption) is not known.

Micronutrients

Zinc

This is an essential trace element used in the formation of proteins and enzymes. The body does not store it and hence on basic principles of poor or inadequate intake in the diet and excessive loss via wounds, burns or the GI tract, it is commonly given to people with wound healing needs. There is some evidence for its role here [15]. Zinc deficiency has also been implicated in disturbed taste activity in elderly people and this too may be part of its effect in the wound healing process [16].

Iron

Iron deficiency anaemia is one of the more common anaemias. It should rarely be ascribed to a poor diet, however, even in elderly people. The most common cause is GI blood loss and in most cases the precise reason should be sought and appropriate treatment given. Other causes of anaemia include the macrocytic ones usually due to vitamin B12 or folic acid deficiency. Normochromic anaemias may be secondary to prolonged chronic diseases including chronic wounds. Anaemia per se seems to affect wound healing with treatment enhancing it. This is probably related to the role of iron in oxygen delivery and collagen synthesis.

Copper

Copper is another essential element within the body and its role is intimately connected to that of iron. Its major roles appear to be in collagen synthesis and in normal white cell production. This is important in deficiency states when there can be neutropaenia (low numbers of white blood cells) and an increased susceptibility to infections.

Vitamin C

This water soluble vitamin is important in many aspects of the wound healing process. Deficiency states are more common in elderly people, especially those in some form of institution. This appears to be related to the dietary intake (less fresh food, poor cooking methods and inadequate intake, especially due to poor dentition). Body stores are not excessive (probably a few months in ideal circumstances) and stores are rapidly used up if an individual is stressed (e.g. injury or infection).

Vitamin C is essential for collagen synthesis and in deficient states the collagen formed has inadequate tensile strength and wounds tend to dehisce (open up, especially postoperatively). It is also essential in blood formation and in deficient states there is in addition capillary fragility which, combined with poor collagen synthesis, leads to less well supported blood vessels and hence excessive bruising and overbleeding. These aspects of vitamin C deficiency have been known and recorded for hundreds of years via the traumatic experiences of sailors. The dramatic cure of scurvy (vitamin C deficiency) with lime juice in this population is also well known.

Nowadays clinical scurvy of such a degree is rare though most medical students know to hunt for the corkscrew hairs with a perifollicular haemorrhage at their base (but never find them!). Subclinical deficiency may be much harder to diagnose. Its measurement is difficult with leucocyte ascorbic acid assays being performed only in some centres and its correlation with deficiency states unclear. Urine testing can be performed with loading doses of vitamin C being given until it appears in the urine (the length of time this takes being some indication of the degree of deficiency). In view of the fact that it is such an essential component in wound healing, especially, it appears, in pressure sores, it is usually given empirically. In addition to the above roles it is also concerned with white blood cell formation (increased risk of infection in deficient states) and it is a powerful antioxidant and hence lessens the damage done to tissues by free radicals. This probably has a long term importance in general tissue integrity as well as a specific role where there is free radical damage, for example during/after tissue ischaemia. This may explain its crucial role in pressure sore damage.

B complex vitamins

These include thiamine (B1), riboflavine (B2), pyridoxine (B6) and cyanocobalamin (B12). In a similar manner to vitamin C, the B complex vitamins are essential for many of the fundamental wound healing processes. They are involved in synthesizing the components for tissue repair, help collagen strength by enhancing the crosslinks and are involved in the immune system and infection control. They too are water soluble.

Vitamin A

This is a fat soluble vitamin whose importance in wound healing is only now being explored. The indications are that it has similar actions to vitamins C and B complex.

Vitamin E

Another fat soluble vitamin, this has achieved some notoriety as one of the fabled elixirs of youth. For many years (and to much derision) some people have advocated it as a general panacea against the ageing process. A leading proponent is Barbara Cartland. The scoffers and pessimists now have to think again as it has been shown that vitamin E is a powerful antioxidant and hence mops up free radicals, the elements in cells that appear to cause cell damage. This may confer specific advantages in wound care as well as general ones bodywide.

NUTRITIONAL INTERVENTION AND WOUND HEALING

All patients with wounds need to have their nutritional status assessed. Preliminary screening by non-experts may be feasible but in certain cases (severe illness, large chronic wounds, poorly healing wounds, burns, inability to take appropriate oral intake) specialist advice is necessary. The dietitian or other member of the nutrition team may use various formulae to estimate the nutritional needs. In addition precise regular weighing of the person should occur as well as an estimation of their current oral intake (fluids and solids) and their previous dietary history. Current medical problems need to be assessed (including the likelihood of improvement or deterioration in their general condition) as well as any special issues (dentition, ethnic nutritional requirements and psychological or psychiatric needs). In addition the person's current and past medication needs to be reviewed for its impact on nutrition in general and wound healing in particular (e.g. steroids and non-steroidal anti-inflammatory drugs – steroids can precipitate diabetes mellitus, mask infection and delay wound healing; NSAIDs predispose to gastric ulceration and also delay wound healing).

The nutritional needs of a person should never be seen in isolation from their total/holistic needs. They form part of the complex puzzle in assessment and indeed part of the treatment but all the other parts are equally as important. If the assessed dietary intake is insufficient to meet the calculated needs (maintenance +/− improvement and repair) then nutritional supplements are needed. Oral supplements are most frequently used but at best ongoing assessment is usually half hearted and in many cases inadequate supplementation is occurring. If the clinical examination and biochemical profile (especially albumin) indicate subnutrition, especially in the case of a large chronic wound, serious consideration should be given to tube feeding.

This should be discussed with the dietitian/nutrition team, client and family (especially if the person is cognitively impaired). Fine-bore nasogastric feeding can be used to supplement oral intake (feeds going through at night) or in debilitated people may temporarily become their main route of nutritional access. Expert advice governs the formulation used (often high-protein lactose-free) and the pump rate (slow to begin with, e.g. 50 ml/hr). In wound healing cases it is rarely necessary to consider gastrostomy (tube inserted into the stomach lumen from outside) though the same principles apply.

In severe malnutrition with difficult to heal wounds or gut absorption problems, the nutrition team may recommend total parenteral nutrition (TPN). This may be considered necessary in the short term as the bowel too has become oedematous and hence adequate absorption is unlikely. All nutrition is given via a central line with specialist monitoring of serum biochemistry. As the person recovers they graduate to nasogastric and then oral feeding. Trace elements must be monitored.

In addition to these nutritional considerations, in cases with large or infected exuding wounds thought should be given to specific supplementation. This often has to be empirical considering the lack of research data. Zinc supplementation is common (220 mg b.d.) though it can cause nausea and be counterproductive. Vitamin C in doses up to 1 gm/day (megadose regimes are controversial) are used though no one knows for how long the supplement should continue, especially in ill individuals. Anaemia should be corrected but in the most appropriate way and only after the cause has been ascertained. Iron deficiency anaemia usually responds to oral iron in chronic cases. Blood transfusion should be reserved for those people bleeding acutely. A macrocytic anaemia (MCV >100) may be due to vitamin B12 or folic acid deficiency (there are many other causes) and will respond to replacement of the appropriate vitamin usually accompanied by iron supplements. The anaemia of chronic disease, normochromic/ normocytic, will not respond to iron therapy. Chronic wounds (which may be the cause) often heal more rapidly and the patient usually feels much better following a blood transfusion to bring the haemoglobin up into the normal range.

Other trace elements or other vitamins may be necessary in individual cases but expert advice is always a good basis for starting treatment. A good review of the common causes for deficiency has been written by McLaren [17].

The circle of wound healing makes the actual role of nutrition difficult to ascertain. We know that it is vital and as the person's nutritional state improves they feel better and begin to eat more. The improved strength allows greater activity so that muscle bulk improves and oedema in all areas lessens. Large wounds become smaller so that more of the nutrition goes into overall improved nutrition rather than repair. The other parts of the cycle, addressing other illness processes, improving oxygenation and muscle and joint flexibility with physiotherapy all help improve appetite and so the wheel turns. A part becomes indistinguishable from the whole. A summary of nutritional assessment methods is given below:

- Clinical examination
- Dietary history
- Anthropometry
- Urinalysis
- Biochemical
- Haematological.

THE AGEING PROCESS AND WOUND HEALING

> We are ignorant of the basic scientific processes underlying wound healing, particularly in the elderly . . . this ignorance and our resulting deficiencies in clinical management means that the majority of wounds are being maintained by nursing and medical care, not cured [18].

These indicting remarks stress the fact that we know comparatively little about the general healing process and even less about the special features that are present in the largest group with chronic wounds, elderly people. The whole area is bedevilled by the problems of ageism both in society in general and the medical and nursing professions in particular. The current textbooks need to be rewritten and the current lectures revamped to accommodate the knowledge base that has been accumulated. The important issues as they affect skin, wounds and elderly people are contained in Chapter 1 and cover areas such as the geriatric giants, Strehler's theories concerning the ageing process, etc. What is known about wound healing and the ageing process can be divided into macro and micro elements. The macro elements involving the whole organism, as it were, and the micro concentrating on some of the known histological and biochemical changes.

At the macro level it is fairly obvious that wounds heal even in very elderly people. The rate of healing may be slower but we cannot be sure of this as the research work has not been done. The problem in this area is still the one of separating the effects of ageing (physiology) from disease (pathology). Elderly people are more likely to have multiple illness processes, take more medication, visit their doctor more frequently and spend longer in hospital or recovering from disease. These facts are not disputed but it makes nonsense of scientific evaluation and research if these same individuals are the ones used to determine wound healing rates. A similar sample of younger people who suffered from chronic disease, e.g. diabetes, renal failure, etc., would show different healing rates yet they would not be considered representative of healthy people in their age group. Work in this area has to be done on health status defined populations to separate out this physiology/pathology effect.

Much of the research work into the ageing process and wound healing is performed on animal models. This may not always be appropriate as there is a lack of a suitable animal model when it comes to chronic wounds, the biggest category of wounds affecting older people. Comparison of healing rates between older and younger human populations is feasible by the increased use of biopsy techniques at various stages of the wound healing process. This is obviously invasive and the cost–benefit aspects would need open discussion yet it would be one way of overcoming some of the animal model difficulties and the advantages could be considerable. Biopsy techniques are becoming far less invasive, painful and costly and this too is a consideration when preparing ethical permission protocols.

At the micro level there have been major advances in cell and molecular biology. The knowledge base is less certain when it comes to the role of antioxidants and free radical damage or in precursor cell biology (the influence of stem cells). Within skin ageing itself we know that the epidermis gets a bit thinner and the dermis alters with reduced amounts of extracellular matrix proteins, collagen and elastin. The thinner epidermis obviously means a diminished barrier function yet the majority of elderly people do not have skin integrity problems. The link with disease and ill health remains crucial. With increasing age there is a much higher risk of photocarcinogenesis in habitually sun exposed and photoaged skin. Ageing skin appears to epithelialize more slowly after injury and there is also an apparent reduction in the skin immunosurveillance system involving Langerhans cells and epidermotrophic T-lymphocytes.

The changes in the dermis may have possible implications for its role with growth factors. It is theorized that the dermis may interact with and stabilize growth factors, providing protection from degradation or long term storage.

The dermis may even interact synergistically with the factors, leading to their increased activity. From the work that has been done on growth factors it seems that donor age appears to influence proliferative capacity and lifespan in culture. With increasing age there is diminished *in vitro* response and impaired growth factor processing by cells. Age also appears to influence growth factor production by cells.

These findings confirm a gradual decline in all wound healing parameters with age but they have to be interpreted cautiously. There is still no good evidence that these changes have any clinical or practical significance except in sick older people (when one should probably expect marked physiological changes). The ageing aspects concerned with wound healing in healthy older populations will hopefully correspond with the other physiological changes currently undergoing investigation and prove to be a declining but benign process, the really important aspects being the possible preventive and interventive roles possible when illness (pathology) occurs.

REFERENCES

1. Silver, I.A. (1980) The physiology of wound healing, in *Wound Healing and Wound Infection* (ed. T.K. Hunt), Appleton Century Crofts, New York, pp. 11–28.
2. Forrester, J.C. (1988) Wound healing and fibrosis, in *Jamieson and Kay's Textbook of Surgical Physiology* (eds I. Ledingham and C. Mackay), Churchill Livingstone, Edinburgh.
3. Champion, R., Burton, J. and Ebling, F. (eds) (1991) *Textbook of Dermatology, Vol. 1*, 5th edn, Blackwell Scientific, Oxford, pp. 219–520.
4. Brown, G.L. *et al.* (1988) Acceleration of tensile strength of incisions treated with EGF and TGF β. *Ann Surg,* **208**, 788–94.
5. McGee, G.S. *et al.* (1988) Recombinant basic fibroblast growth factor accelerates wound healing. *J Surg Res,* **45**, 145–53.
6. Gabbiani, G. (1981) The myofibroblast: a key cell for wound healing and fibrocontractive diseases. *Progress Clin Biol Res,* **54**, 183–94.
7. Hunt, T.K., Zederfeldt, B. and Goldstick, T.K. (1969) Oxygen and healing. *Am J Surg,* **118**, 521–5.
8. Knighton, D.R., Thakral, K.K. and Hunt, T.K. (1980) Platelet derived angiogenesis initiator of the healing sequence. *Surg Forum* **31**, 226–7.
9. Allen, M.W. (1992) Hyperbaric oxygen therapy – a new wound treatment? *Wound Man,* **2**, 6.
10. Sporn, M.B. and Roberts, A.B. (1988) Peptide growth factors are multi functional. *Nature,* **32**, 217–19.
11. Glover, M. (1992) Growth factors and wound healing. *Wound Man,* **2**(1), 9–11.
12. Detsky, A.S. and Baker, J.P. (1987) Perioperative nutrition: a meta-analysis of the literature. *Ann Int Med,* **107**, 195–203.
13. Gregory, J., Foster, K., Tyler, H.O. and Wiseman, M. (1990) *The Dietary and Nutritional Survey of British Adults,* OPCS/HMSO, London.
14. Durnin, J.V.G.A. and Lean, M.E.J. (1992) Nutrition – considerations for the elderly, in *Textbook of Geriatric Medicine and Gerontology,* 4th edn, (eds J. C. Brocklehurst, R.C. Tallis and H.M. Fillit), Churchill Livingstone, Edinburgh.

15. Pories, W.J. *et al.* (1967) Acceleration of wound healing in man with zinc sulphate. *Lancet*, **i**, 121–4.
16. Sandstead, H.H., Henrickson, L.K., Greger, J.L., Prasas, A.S. and Good, R.A. (1982) Zinc nutriture in the elderly in relation to taste activity, immune response and wound healing. *AMJ Clin Nutr*, **36**, 1046–59.
17. McLaren, S. (1993) Nutritional factors in wound healing. *Wound Man*, **3**(1), 8–10.
18. Ferguson, M. (1993) Paper presented at the Wound Healing and Ageing Workshop, King's Fund Centre, London, 2 March.

The holistic approach to wound assessment
3

Assessment is an integral part of the wound management process and should reflect a holistic and multidisciplinary team approach to patient care.

Holism is a philosophical theory belonging to the system of biological thought. In the context of nursing, holism relates to the whole person and the importance of understanding the complexity of that person and how the different components of that individual influence their life. Its successful application to nursing is dependent on the practitioner's ability to systematically collect, assimilate, record and utilize relevant patient information [1], thereby enabling effective planning and care to be delivered by ensuring that opportunities for intervention are not missed or complications arising from underlying pathology overlooked.

A FRAMEWORK FOR ASSESSMENT

Nursing practice is constantly evolving as nurses endeavour to meet the changing demands society makes on the professional. In the last three decades nursing models have been created; these form a logical framework on which to base nursing interventions and actions [2]. This chapter provides the reader with a broad assessment framework based on a model of activities of living [3] and self-care [4] which enables assessment to be viewed as an ongoing process.

The first concept [3] for discussion has 12 activities of living as its central focus for assessment, each activity being considered in the context of a biological, developmental and social dimension.

The 12 activities are:

1. maintaining a safe environment
2. controlling body temperature
3. communication
4. mobilizing
5. breathing
6. personal hygiene and dressing
7. working and playing
8. eating and drinking
9. expressing sexuality
10. eliminating
11. sleeping
12. dying.

The central focus for nursing intervention is based upon the assessment findings and gives consideration to five key components:

1. activities of living;
2. patient lifespan;
3. degree of patient dependence/independence;
4. factors influencing activities of living;
5. individuality in living and nursing intervention.

Every aspect of living is influenced by the process of physical, intellectual, emotional and social development which occurs throughout life [3]. Part of the nursing assessment is to reflect on the stage of development the patient has currently reached and its influence on the nursing intervention.

A person's ability to perform activities of living independently is assessed on a dependence/independence continuum and enables the practitioner to take account of changes in a person's dependency that can occur throughout their lifespan and for numerous reasons. It is the effects of a change in dependency that practitioners need to consider when deciding with the patient or their carers on the type and level of nursing intervention.

Five key factors thought to influence the activities of living have been identified [3]:

1. physical
2. psychological
3. politicoeconomic
4. sociocultural
5. environmental.

It is not within the scope of this text to discuss models of nursing in depth. The intention is to highlight the dynamic nature of nursing and to give recognition to the concept that nursing may be viewed as helping patients to prevent, solve, alleviate or cope with the problems associated with the activities of daily living. The importance of individualized nursing based on the holistic assessment of needs requires the application of critical thinking skills. Good clinical practice arises from the practitioner's ability to identify and prioritize care requirements with the patient and/or their carers.

The development of the care plan should, where appropriate, involve other members of the multidisciplinary team. Where care is to be on a shared basis or involving other agencies, all parties must have a clear understanding of their role in the provision of care. When the delegation of care is to lay carers or junior members of the team, their ability to fulfil the care requirements safely and competently must be ascertained.

All programmes of care should be monitored and evaluated to assess their effectiveness in achieving the management objectives or outcomes.

One of the key components of care is the ability of the nurse to recognize and respect the uniqueness and dignity of each patient and respond to their need for care [5]. Orem's philosophy when applied to wound care is concerned with the ability of the individual to maintain a delicate balance between the demands made upon them by their general state of health, presence of a wound and their self-care abilities. Orem suggests that an individual needs sufficient self-care ability to meet six universal self-care demands and cope with illness. These abilities are defined as:

1. having sufficient intake of air, food and water;
2. satisfactorily eliminating waste products;
3. maintaining a balance between activity and rest;
4. being aware of and preventing danger or hazard to self;
5. maintaining a balance between solitude and social interaction;
6. maintaining normalcy.

The presence of a wound can provoke a major change in an individual's lifestyle due to physical, psychological or social factors that result in a deficit between self-care demand and self-care ability.

Chronic wounds, in particular those associated with underlying malignancy or acute wounds that result in extensive tissue loss and altered body image, can have a profound effect upon an individual and their family.

RATIONALE FOR INTERVENTION

The assessment process should seek to establish the level and rationale for intervention. In many situations care is on a shared basis between relevant members of the multidisciplinary team, the patient and their carers. It must always be remembered that some wounds are very dynamic and their characteristics can change dramatically over a short period of time, hence the need for effective communication and good record keeping. Three approaches to intervention, reflecting different levels of self-care ability [4] are proposed:

1. educative/supportive;
2. partly compensatory;
3. wholly compensatory.

The educative/supportive approach provides a framework for both patient and nurse. The nurse uses teaching and communication skills to assist the patient through the acquisition of knowledge, skill and confidence to attain an optimum level of self-care and hence maintain patient independence. This is especially important for patients with leg ulcers to facilitate healing and to avoid reulceration or for patients whose wounds are complex or difficult to heal or require palliative management.

With the partly compensatory approach the nursing intervention focuses on promoting self-care, while compensating for identified self-care deficits.

The wholly compensatory approach is directed towards the patient whose condition leaves them with little or no self-care ability.

The absence of the ability to maintain a balance between self-care ability and self-care demand [6] validates the need for nursing intervention. Nursing intervention may therefore consist of giving guidance or teaching the patient to practise self-care, assisting the patient or carrying out the task entirely for the patient [7], depending upon self-care needs and self-care ability. Many patients with either chronic or acute wounds may experience one or more intervention approaches.

THE ASSESSMENT PROCESS

The value of the nursing assessment to the patient is determined by the skill of the nurse. The information relevant to the identification of the patient's needs may be difficult to extrapolate especially if the patient has, for whatever reason, gone to great lengths to conceal the problem from relatives or friends. The patient's willingness to communicate may also relate to their level of acceptance of their disease and prognosis. Problems in communicating may also arise due to cultural differences, speech or hearing impediments or other dysfunctions.

PATIENT RECORDS

The importance of adopting a multidisciplinary approach to patient assessment is an integral part of the holistic process.

The need to give due consideration to all the relevant factors influencing wound healing is an essential component for effective care. By commencing with a broad data base, the effectiveness of local

Name _____ Weight _____ Date _____

Please tick if patient is having a portion of the following foods for each serving.

Food groups	Breakfast	Mid-morning	Mid-day	Afternoon	Evening meal	During evening/ bedtime	No. of servings	
							Total	Target
Starchy foods Breakfast cereal Bread Biscuits/cakes Pudding (not milk) Pasta/rice								6 for MEN or 5 for WOMEN
Fruit & vegetables Vegetables Salad Fruit Fruit juice Potato								3
Protein foods Baked beans Meat/fish Poultry Egg Cheese Milk pudding/ custard								5 FOR MEN OR 4 FOR WOMEN
Milky drinks Coffee/malted Milk Drinks made with ALL milk								
Supplements eg. Complan (Please name)								8 CUPS
Other beverages Soup/Bovril Tea/coffee Squash/water Beers, etc.								
Comments Relevant to patient's intake								

Figure 3.1 Nutritional check list. Adapted from work undertaken in the Bournemouth and Christchurch NHS Trust.

Notes to help you complete the nutritional check list

Please put one tick in the appropriate box when food is eaten.

1. *Bread*
   - One tick for one whole slice. Please write ½ in box if only ½ slice eaten. Please put 2 ticks (✔ ✔) if 2 slices eaten (as in one whole round of sandwiches).
   - Sandwiches - put ticks for bread AND the filling separately.

2. *Biscuits*
   - Include crackers or crispbread.

3. *Puddings*
   - Include pastry, crumble, sponge, jelly, ice cream, mousse.

4. *Milk puddings*
   - Includes custard. So fruit and custard or pie and custard will get a tick in 2 different boxes.

5. *Cheese*
   - This would get a tick for a cheese dish such as cauliflower cheese or macaroni cheese or cheese sandwich or cheese and biscuits. All these items will also get a tick in another box (for the pasta, bread, crackers or veg.).

6. *Milky drinks*
   - Includes all drinks made with all milk such as coffee, Horlicks, Ovaltine, plain milk. If ½ cup had (e.g. half milk, half water coffee) write ½.

7. *Fluids*
   - This includes all other beverages such as tea, coffee made without much milk, Bovril, squash, water, alcoholic drink. Also soup (as this does not have much nutritive value).

8. *Supplements*
   - e.g. Complan, Fortisip.

9. *Comments*
   - Note if on fluid or puréed food only. Also note under here if sugar is taken in drinks and if sweets or chocolates have been eaten.

If you do not think this intake was fairly typical please state why.

Figure 3.1 *continued*

wound management programmes can be objectively and frequently evaluated and unnecessary changes to the treatment programme avoided.
The following are offered as general points for consideration:

GENERAL HEALTH CONSIDERATIONS

- Respiratory function
- Cardiovascular status
- Sensory function
- Skin appearance
- Self-care ability
- Presence or absence of pain
- Current medication
- Mobility
- Type of home environment
- Sleep pattern
- Patient's expectations/priorities
- Mental alertness
- Level of consciousness
- Emotional status
- Immune status
- Allergies
- Social circumstances
- Lifestyle
- Continence
- Social contacts
- Nutritional status
- Adjuvant therapy
- Patient's understanding of present condition and prognosis
- Multidisciplinary team's expectations/priorities
- Type of intervention: active to promote healing, palliative to treat symptoms

As highlighted in Chapter 2, wound healing and tissue integrity can be greatly enhanced or compromised by dietary intake, absorption and utilization of fluid and nutrients. The term 'malnutrition' is widely used but there exists no internationally accepted definition of the malnourished state [8] and many patients do not even have a basic assessment of their nutritional status. Despite advances in our knowledge of nutrition and wound healing over the past decade and continuing professional interest, further research is necessary to determine how best to manipulate dietary intake in order to ensure an optimal supply of nutrient substrates to the infiltrate, whilst meeting general metabolic requirements [9].

Wound metabolism is to a great extent governed by a local cellular infiltrate. Following injury, glucose provides a vital energy substrate for cellular infiltration of leucocytes and macrophages, both of which have a high capacity for aerobic glycolysis and a crucial role in the production of factors which stimulate fibroblast growth and collagen synthesis. Early nutritional assessment is essential to ascertain the patient's dietary requirements and method of attainment [10].

DIETARY HISTORY

Obtaining a dietary history, whilst appearing relatively easy, can lead to inappropriate information being collected as it is dependent upon the memory recall of the patient and their willingness to declare dietary intake. Even observation and recording of dietary intake for hospital or residential care patients can result in omissions. Ideally patients considered to be malnourished or at least at risk of malnutrition should have their dietary intake recorded for each 24 hours over a period of seven to 28 days. All high risk patients should have a weighed intake at least every third day. Information on actual intake can then be compared with the recommended daily requirements. A simple dietary intake checklist (Figure 3.1) and method of calculating the patient's daily dietary intake should be readily available and used by all practitioners. The need for the early involvement of the dietitian should be clearly recognized and a referral system implemented in every health district.

The primary aims of nutritional support are to maintain lean body mass and organ function, promote healing, improve immunocompetence and thereby reduce morbidity and mortality associated with a disorder and its treatment [11]. For additional information on nutrition and wound healing, please refer to the references and recommended reading.

Table 3.1 Possible responses to a painful event

Resolution	Medical solution Elimination of pain
Adaption	Nursing solution Adaption of pain and life events
Maladaptation	Maladaptive behavioural responses which impede recovery
Resistance	Search for pain control and unwillingness to adapt to pain
Depression	Total loss of control

PAIN ASSESSMENT

The need for a comprehensive assessment of pain and its impact on the quality of the patient's life and wound management programme is frequently neglected.

Pain from whatever cause is almost always associated with an unpleasant experience and its dynamic and complex nature can prove a significant challenge to both medical and nursing practitioners.

Acute pain can be characterized by a combination of factors and includes tissue damage, pain and anxiety associated with hyperactivity of the sympathetic nervous system. It may be a warning sign for impending actual physical damage. By contrast chronic benign pain may represent a complex biopsychosocial phenomenon [13].

The impact of inadequate pain assessment and lack of professional support or empathy has been highlighted [13] and includes loss of sleep, frustration, irritability and anger, loss of appetite, muscle tension and anxiety, increasing dependence, social isolation, altered mental status and depression. A study of elderly patients [13] with pain identified possible responses to painful stimuli (Table 3.1), the importance of the nurse's role in the psychological management of persistent intractable pain and the need for a systematic approach to assessment and intervention. This view is based on the premise that coping with pain is dependent upon a wide range of different factors, but that active coping is the most adaptive. Concrete ways in which the nurse can fulfil the patient's emotional needs with respect to pain management are summarized in Figure 3.2.

WOUND ASSESSMENT

A comprehensive and accurate assessment of the patient's wound and surrounding tissue is essential for critical evaluation of the wound

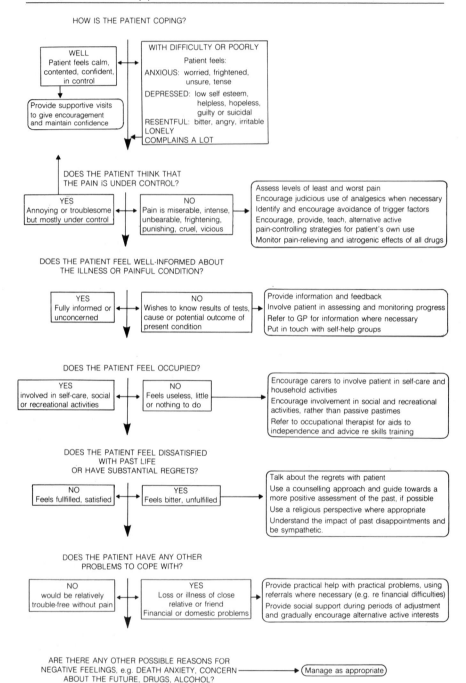

Figure 3.2 The nursing management of elderly patients with pain, in the community. Adapted with kind permission from [13].

healing process and management regime. Failure to accurately assess and clearly document relevant information can result in the practitioner being held legally, ethically and morally accountable for inadequacies in the patient's nursing management. Baseline information may include:

- date and time injury/wound occurred (if known);
- aetiology/cause of the wound;
- location and extent of tissue damage;
- dimension of the wound;
- wound characteristics;
- anticipated method of healing.

Local factors considered adverse to the healing process or palliative care:

- clinical infection
- necrotic tissue
- slough
- odour
- pain
- poor perfusion
- oedema
- excessive exudate.

Characteristics of surrounding tissues:

- healthy
- macerated
- dry/flaky
- eczema
- blue/black discolouration
- oedema
- erythema
- cellulitis.

The presence of clinically infected tissue gives rise to several well recognized and documented findings including inflamed, hot, swollen, painful tissues with or without the presence of pus. It is generally advisable to identify the cause of the infection and establish the antibiotics to which the organism is sensitive. Suspicion of a clinical infection is justification for swabbing the wound; it is important to reassure the patient and explain the procedure before commencing this activity. All the necessary equipment should be assembled before the wound is exposed and care taken to avoid self or swab contamination. The swab should be taken from the edge of the wound as this is an area of high tissue activity, but avoiding the surrounding skin.

Wherever possible, collect the specimen before antibiotics have been taken. Always note on the form if the patient has had a course of antibiotics and what they were. Sufficient clinical information must always be provided to the laboratory staff. It is insufficient to state 'leg ulcer' or 'pressure sores'. Most departments have guidelines on the information required. The provision of good quality information will prevent unnecessary expenditure.

Location of Wound(s)   (Please circle appropriate response)

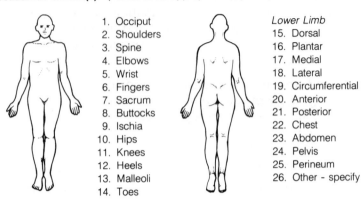

1. Occiput	*Lower Limb*
2. Shoulders	15. Dorsal
3. Spine	16. Plantar
4. Elbows	17. Medial
5. Wrist	18. Lateral
6. Fingers	19. Circumferential
7. Sacrum	20. Anterior
8. Buttocks	21. Posterior
9. Ischia	22. Chest
10. Hips	23. Abdomen
11. Knees	24. Pelvis
12. Heels	25. Perineum
13. Malleoli	26. Other - specify
14. Toes	

Type of wound

Date .... Location............. Duration	Date .... Location .... Duration	Date .... Location .... Duration
Wound bed Healthy epithelium Granulation slough necrotic (hard/soft)	**Wound bed** Healthy epithelium Granulation slough necrotic (hard/soft)	**Wound bed** Healthy epithelium Granulation slough necrotic (hard/soft)
Clinical infection swab sent Suspected/confirmed/ no sign	Suspected/confirmed/ no sign	Suspected/confirmed/ no sign
Exudate discharge type Blood/pus/serum	Blood/pus/serum	Blood/pus/serum
Exudate discharge Clear/pink/dark red/green/ light red/pinky yellow/ other	Clear/pink/dark red/green/ light red/pinky yellow/ other	Clear/pink/dark red/green/ light red/pinky yellow/ other ....
Amount None/slight/moderate/heavy	None/slight/moderate/heavy	None/slight/moderate/heavy
Odour None/some/offensive	None/some/offensive	none/some/offensive
Wound edges Healthy, oedematous Red/pink/purple/yellow/ green/black other	Healthy, oedematous Red/pink/purple/yellow/ green/black other	healthy, oedematous Red/pink/purple/yellow/ green/black other ....
Surrounding skin Red/pink/purple/pale/blue/ black/macerated/healthy/ eczema cellulitis	Red/pink/purple/pale/blue/ black/macerated/healthy/ eczema	Red/pink/purple/pale/blue/ black/macerated/healthy/ eczema
Oedema of surrounding skin Present/not present	Present/not present	Present/not present
Photograph Measured Size of wound	Photograph Measured Size of wound	Photograph Measured Size of wound
Pain - wound site None 0, Slight <3, Moderate 4-6, Severe 7-10, Continuous, Intermittent	None 0, Slight <3, Moderate 4-6, Severe 7-10, Continuous, Intermittent	None 0, Slight <3, Moderate 4-6, Severe 7-10, Continuous, Intermittent ....

Figure 3.3 Wound assessment/prescription chart.

Patient name Address DOB Hospital No.	Hospital Dept/ward Consultant Known allergies

Summary of treatment programme – review at least weekly

Prescription required					Pharmacy	
Product	Size	Amount	Signature	Date for review	Dispensed	Signature of pharmacist

Dressings Prescribed by:
Registered Nurse

Kaltostat	7.5 × 12 cm 15 × 25 cm	10 × 20 cm 5 × 5
Kaltostat Cavity	2g	
Lyofoam	10 × 10 cm	20 × 15 cm
Comfeel Transparent	5 × 7 cm 15 × 20 cm	9 × 14 cm
Comfeel Ulcer	10 × 10 cm 20 × 20 cm	15 × 15 cm
Comfeel Paste	50 g	
IntraSite Gel	15 g	25 g
Jelonet	5 × 5 cm 10 × 40 cm 15 cm × 2 m	10 × 10 cm 10 × 7 cm
Granuflex Thin	10 × 10 cm	7.5 × 7.5 cm
Granuflex Border	6 × 6 cm 13 × 15 cm	10 × 10 cm 18 × 20 cm

Consultant or Nurse Specialist

Kaltostat Fortex	7.5 × 12 cm	15 × 15 cm
Kaltocarb	10 × 10 cm	15 × 20 cm
Allevyn	10 × 10 cm	20 × 20 cm
Comfeel Pressure Relieving Dressing	10 × 7 cm 15 × 15 cm	10 × 10 cm
Spenco 2nd Skin Spenco Dermal Pad	5 × 7.5 cm	7.5 × 10 cm
Iodosorb	10 g	
Iodoflex	5 g	10 g
Tegapore	7.5 × 10 cm	20 × 20 cm
Mepitel	5 × 7.5 cm 18 × 10 cm	7.5 × 10 cm 20 × 30 cm
Paste bandages		
Silastic foam		
1% metronidazole in gel		

Figure 3.3 *continued*

PRINCIPLES FOR OBTAINING AND HANDLING A SPECIMEN

- All containers should be labelled in advance.
- Take care not to contaminate the outside of the container by touching it with the swab or with a 'dirty' gloved hand.
- The swab should reach the laboratory as soon as possible after collection while it is still moist. If a delay is unavoidable, the specimen should be placed in a sterile moist broth to preserve its viability.

Some laboratories prefer all swabs to be transported in a culture medium. If you are unsure, contact the laboratory and ask for advice. Ensure that the form is completed accurately. As well as the patient's details, it should show the site from where the swab was taken. The nature of the wound should be described [14]. (For further information please see references 15, 16 and 17).

The following wounds may require specialist assessment because of the potential complications:

- penetrating wounds;
- potentially disfiguring wounds of the face;
- suspected non-accidental injuries;
- difficult to remove foreign bodies;
- crush injuries;
- non-superficial burns/scalds.

WOUND MEASUREMENT

Methods of measuring wound dimensions range from using complex equipment to a simple linear tracing. The use of a double layer of domestic clear film enables the wound contact layer to be discarded. The top layer can be filed in the patient's notes for future reference and comparison of wound size. Additional information may include the length and direction of existing sinuses and location of different wound characteristics. Many companies now provide cards and pens for tracing and measuring wounds free of charge.

The depth of a wound may be measured by using a gloved finger, spatula or probe. A ruler or measuring device may be placed over the surface of the wound and a probe gently passed down to the wound base. On removal the distance between the tip of the probe and skin surface is measured. For irregular shaped cavities the procedure can be repeated at regular intervals along the wound bed. Practitioners need to be particularly careful when investigating the direction and length of suspected sinus tracts so as not to damage the delicate tissues. It is advisable to photograph most complicated or chronic wounds (malignant fungatings wounds may be one exception), thereby providing more objective evidence of surface area changes and thus complementing the written description.

CONCLUSION

Assessment forms the basis from which a patient's care needs are identified and is the key to successful intervention. The time and place of assessment has a direct bearing on its value; effective planning and delivery of nursing care can only be achieved if a comprehensive patient assessment is undertaken and is based on this nursing plan and all future reassessment which will follow while the patient is receiving care, whether in hospital or community [18].

On completion of the assessment process the practitioner should have sufficient information about the patient and their situation to make an informed judgement of the patient's general health, wound characteristics and factors which may influence the healing process.

The method used by practitioners to document their assessment findings will inevitably vary in design, although some of the information to be recorded will be similar irrespective of wound aetiology (Figure 3.3).

The practitioner must now consider what would constitute appropriate/acceptable wound management.

REFERENCES

1. Moody, M. and Grocott, P. (1993) *A Practical Approach to the Holistic Management of Patients with Fungating Malignant Wounds*. Booklet published for study day organized by *Professional Nurse*, available from the authors.
2. Moody, M. (1990) *Incontinence in Patient Problems and Nursing Care*, Heinemann Nursing, Oxford.
3. Roper, N. Logan, W. and Tierney, A. (1985) *The Elements of Nursing*, Churchill Livingstone, London.
4. Orem, D. (1985) *Nursing: Concepts of Practice*, 3rd edn, McGraw-Hill, New York.
5. United Kingdom Central Council (1992) *Code of Professional Conduct for the Nurse, Midwife and Health Visitor*, 3rd edn, UKCC, London.
6. Orem, D. (1991) *Nursing: Concepts of Practice*, 4th edn, Mosby, St. Louis.
7. Pearson, A. and Vaughan, B. (1986) *Nursing Models for Practice*, Heinemann, London.
8. Ingerslev, J. (1992) 'Nutrition, age and wound healing in theory, in *Advanced Wound Healing Resource Pack*, (ed. K. Harting), Coloplast (UK), Peterborough.
9. McLaren Goodison, S. (1993) 'Nutrition factors in wound healing: theoretical considerations, wound management. *Nurse*, 3(1), 8–10.

10. McLaren Goodison, S. (1993) Nutritional support in wound care 2: assessment techniques and nutrient requirements. *Wound Man*, **4**(1), 31–4.
11. Moody, M. (1992) 'Problem wounds: a nursing challenge.' RCN Nursing Update. *Nursing Standard*, **7**(6), 3–8.
12. Dickenson, J.W.T. and Wright, J. (1986) Hospital induced malnutrition, in *Nutrition in Nursing Practice*, (ed. S. Holmes), University of Surrey, Guildford.
13. Walker, J.M. (1989) 'The management of elderly patients with pain: a community nursing perspective.' Doctoral thesis, Nursing and Health Care Research Unit, Dorset Institute of Higher Education (now Institute of Health and Community Services), University of Bournemouth, published as Walker, J.M. (1990) [title as above]. *Journal of Advanced Nursing*, **15**, 1160.
14. Cheesman, S. (1992) Taking a wound swab, in *A Pocket Guide to Wound Management*, (ed. M. Moody), Dorset and Salisbury College of Midwifery and Nursing (now part of the Institute of Health and Community Services), University of Bournemouth.
15. Kee, J.L. (1983) *Laboratory and Diagnostic Tests with Nursing Implications*, Appleton Century Crofts, New York.
16. Bushall, A.C. (1989) Bacteriology of superficial and deep tissue infection, in *Medical Bacteriology*, (ed. P.M. Hawkey and D.A. Lewis), IAK Press, Oxford, pp. 91–137.
17. Lawrence, J.C. (1993) Wound colonisation and infection with particular reference to burns and chronic wounds, in *Advanced Wound Healing Resource Pack*, (ed. K. Harting), Coloplast (UK), Peterborough.
18. Feely, M. (1994) Know your patient: the importance of assessment in care delivery. *Prof Nurse*, **9**(5), 318–23

Principles of wound management

4

A key component of care is the nurse's ability to recognize and respect the uniqueness and dignity of each patient and to respond to their need for care [1].

Effective wound management is based on the application of principles for good practice. On completion of the holistic assessment the nurse must make an informed judgement which reflects their analysis of the patient's general health, wound characteristics and factors which may influence the healing process. Wherever possible the patient and/or their carers should be part of the decision making process. Factors for consideration include issues of acceptability and appropriateness of the proposed plan of action. For example, is the dressing:

- acceptable to the patient?
- suitable for the current stage of healing?
- of an acceptable quality?
- cost effective?
- appropriate for the care environment?
- available?

There now exists a considerable body of knowledge to explain many of the highly complex biochemical and metabolic processes involved in wound healing. This knowledge, when combined with information and research findings on wound dressing products, can assist the nurse to select a product which will enhance the creation of an optimum microenvironment for rapid and pain-free tissue repair.

It is therefore necessary for the nurse to know:

- what wound products are available;
- what the claimed performance is;

- how and when the product should be used;
- duration of use;
- the tissue's normal and abnormal response.

The ability to select an appropriate wound dressing is therefore an integral part of the nurse's role in assisting the wound healing process [2].

Considerable progress has been made since the development in 1880 of the 'Gamgee Pad' by Joseph Gamgee. The traditional acceptance of an absorbent wound cover which frequently produced a dry surface with problems of adhesion and subsequent trauma has been (generally) replaced by the philosophy that a moist wound is a healing wound [3]. The principle of moist wound healing was first demonstrated by Winter [4].

A number of performance parameters were considered necessary [3] if an acceptable microenvironment was to be both produced and maintained (Table 4.1). Over time these parameters have been modified. Fairbrother suggested that we separate the primary considerations of product efficiency from those of convenience and cost [5]. (Tables 4.2 and 4.3).

Table 4.1 Performance parameters of wound dressings (adapted from [26])

A dressing should have the ability to:

- remove excess exudate and toxic components
- maintain high humidity at the wound/dressing interface
- allow gaseous exchange
- provide thermal insulation
- afford protection from secondary infection
- be free from toxic contaminants
- allow removal without trauma at dressing change

Table 4.2 Dressing performance characteristics: primary considerations ([5])

- Effects on rate and quality of healing
- Bacterial barrier
- Rate and capacity of absorption of exudate
- Occlusivity/gas permeability
- Cytocompatibility
- Hypo-allergenicity
- Wound contact/release characteristics
- Thermal insulation

Table 4.3 Reasons for primary and secondary considerations

Primary consideration	• Optimize wound healing • Prevent infection • Control exudate
Secondary consideration	• Improve quality of life • Improve comfort and convenience • Control odour • Reduce pain and pruritus
Secondary consideration for nursing staff	• Minimize nursing time/ effort • Optimize treatment cost

WOUND DRESSINGS

The ideal dressing should provide an environment at the surface of the wound in which healing may take place at the maximum rate consistent with the production of a healed wound with an acceptable cosmetic appearance [6].

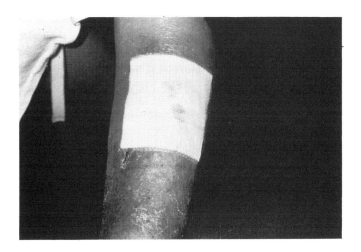

Figure 4.1 Example of a non-absorbent dressing.

PRIMARY CONTACT LOW OR NON-ABSORBENT DRESSINGS

There is a large range of dressings which are classified under this heading so for ease of reference they have been subdivided.

Paraffin tulle gras

Since tulle gras was first introduced during World War 1, there have been several varieties of medicated and non-medicated tulle dressings developed. Traditionally the dressings have been used on superficial or partial thickness wounds. The greasy nature of these dressings combined with their tendency to sometimes cause maceration of the surrounding skin and adherence to the wound can be a problem. Practitioners should also be aware of the potential problems associated with using medicated products due to the variable efficiency of these dressings. The sticky residue remaining on the skin and wound is often difficult to remove. Although cheap to purchase, the necessity for frequent dressing changes combined with the need for a secondary dressing, nursing time required and risk of patient sensitivity must be taken into account before prescribing these products. Hence their therapeutic value must be questioned.

Impregnated viscose

These dressings are impregnated with antimicrobial agents such as 10% povidone iodine in a water based polyethylene glycol base, i.e. Inadine (Johnson & Johnson) which is an orange-brown colour when applied to a wound but goes cream or white to indicate it is time to replace the dressing.

This type of dressing can be used prophylactically or to treat a wide range of bacterial, protozoal and fungal organisms. Despite the low amount of free iodine available some patients may develop a sensitivity. Practitioners must follow the manufacturer's instructions and recommendations for use precisely. Monitoring the efficiency of the dressing can be difficult unless a film dressing is used.

Non-impregnated, non/low adherent dressing

A number of dressings have been produced which contain an absorbent dressing pad. Melolin (Smith & Nephew) has been in use since the late 1960s. Nurses are aware that Melolin does have a tendency to adhere to the wound and that care should be exercised when removing an adherent dressing. Other absorbent low adherent and comfortable dressings include Release (Johnson & Johnson) [7] and Telfa (Robinsons).

Other products such as Silicone NA (Johnson & Johnson) and Mepitel (Mölnlycke) contain silicone and can remain *in situ* without adherence to the wound for up to seven days. This type of dressing is especially useful for delicate and fragile tissue, where dressing changes need to be kept to the absolute minimum, such as:

- burns;
- fixation of grafts;
- painful wounds (finger tip injuries, nail bed surgery);
- weak or sensitive skin (diabetics, radiotherapy patients, steroidal skin);
- leg ulcers;
- abrasions;
- traumatic wounds;
- around joints;
- problem solving – around pin sites, fixation of intravenous cannulae;
- dermatology (epidermolysis bullosa).

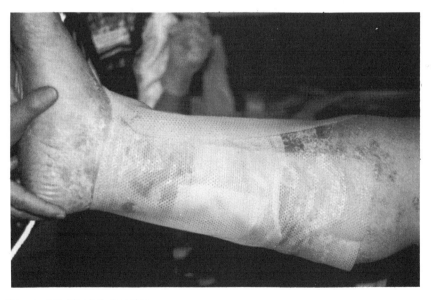

Figure 4.2 Mepitel dressing.

Mepitel is a sterile non-adhesive dressing made of a medical grade silicone gel bound to a soft and pliable polymide net. It will not adhere to the wound yet will adhere to itself and surrounding healthy skin, making it easy to apply.

Tegapore is another non-adherent dressing that can remain *in situ* for seven days. It is made of hypoallergenic polymide and becomes transparent when moist, providing an optimum healing environment.

SEMIPERMEABLE FILM DRESSINGS

There are several film dressings currently available, including Cutifilm (BDF), Opsite (Smith & Nephew), Spyroflex (Britcair), Tegaderm (3M), Bioclusive (Johnson & Johnson) and Spyrosorb (Britcair) (Figure 4.3). Most have a protective outer layer which appears to act as a barrier to bacterial invasion. Film dressings are suitable for superficial and shallow wounds, as a secondary dressing for low adherent products and prophylactically to prevent or reduce skin friction.

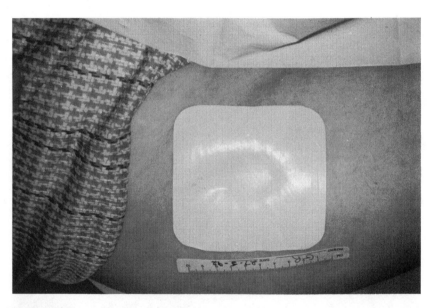

Figure 4.3 Spyrosorb film dressing.

Practitioners should be aware of the importance manufacturers attach to the application and removal of these dressings and that the physical characteristics of the different films have a direct influence th-ir clinical performance.

v of six film dressings undertaken by Thomas *et al.* [8] iden-
najor performance parameters which had a direct influence
performance of the dressing:

1. moisture vapour permeability;
2. tissue compatibility;
3. extensibility of film;
4. weight of film;
5. thickness of film.

FOAM DRESSINGS

Foam dressings were first used for the management of wounds in the 1970s. Silastic foam is a two-component product that forms a foam stent when the base product is mixed with a stannous oxalate catalyst. The stent is removed from the wound cavity for cleaning twice a day and one stent may be used for a week or even longer depending upon the healing process of the wound.

Following a report in 1987 [9] questioning the biological efficiency of some of the chemicals used in the manufacture of plastics, concerns over this dressing were raised. However, all current available evidence indicates that Silastic foam poses no significant risk to the patient and the dressing continues to be a very useful cavity wound filler in many clinical situations.

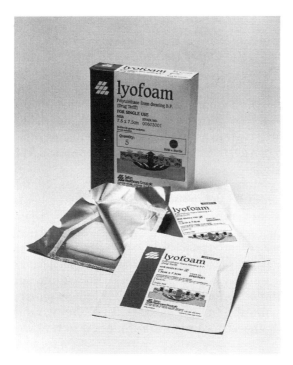

Figure 4.4 Lyofoam dressings.

Lyofoam, a two-layer polyurethane dressing, was also developed in the 1970s as a wound management product. The outer layer of the dressing is hydrophobic and non-absorbent while the layer at the wound interface is smooth, hydrophilic and absorbent. Lyofoam is available on FP10 and may be used on wounds of medium to high exudation. The dressing can be left *in situ* for up to seven days. Variations include Lyofoam A, a polyurethane foam island dressing which requires no secondary dressing, and Lyofoam C which contains activated carbon and has been specially formulated to combat offensive odours.

Allevyn and Allevyn cavity wound dressings both consist of a hydrocellular/hydrophilic polyurethane structure designed to absorb large volumes of exudation. The dressing is highly versatile and can be easily cut and shaped to fit difficult wounds. The polyurethane backing prevents strike-through. It is especially useful for use on moderate to heavy exuding wounds and can be used under compression bandages. Removal is usually easy and completely trauma-free. The cavity dressings are available in four sizes and may be left *in situ* for 4–5 days depending on the amount of exudate.

ALGINATES

Alginates are manufactured from brown seaweed collected off the shores of Ireland, the Outer Hebrides and other coastal parts of the world. The naturally occurring alginic acid consists of a polymer containing varying proportions of mannuronic and guluronic acid residues, depending upon the location and type of seaweed used. Alginates rich in mannuronic acid (Sorbsan) form soft flexible gels while those rich in guluronic acid (Kaltostat) form a much firmer gel. The formation of a gel facilitates an atraumatic removal from the wound bed (Figure 4.5).

Alginate dressings have haemostatic properties [10] initiated by the exchange of sodium ions in the blood and are suitable for a range of moderate to heavy exuding wounds.

The introduction of an alginate cavity filler has greatly enhanced the management of cavity wounds especially when used in conjunction with an effective secondary dressing such as Allevyn or Spyrosorb [11]. The hydrophilic gel that forms across the wound surface enables a pain and trauma-free removal whilst providing a moist environment for healing. Fibres that are embodied in the wound matrix are biodegradable, thereby eliminating the need to remove all traces of the dressing.

Frequency of dressing changes is determined by the uptake of exudate and may vary from daily at first extending to seven days.

Practitioners should be aware of the clinical indication, selection and dressing change criteria for each type of alginate available [11].

Studies demonstrate a high level of patient acceptance. The formation of a gel and subsequent painless dressing change have been shown to reduce the need for analgesia prior to dressing change [12,13].

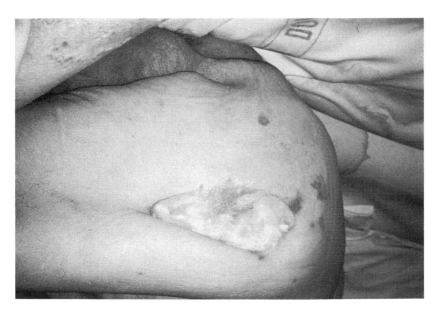

Figure 4.5 Alginate dressing.

HYDROGELS

Hydrogels may be described as insoluble hydrophilic polymers with the capacity to interact at the wound interface to absorb and retain large quantities of fluid.

There are two main types of hydrogels, classified according to whether or not they change their physical form as they absorb fluid. Amorphous hydrogels like Bard Absorption Dressing and IntraSite gradually lose their cohesiveness as they absorb fluid so these changes in viscosity enable the dressing to fill the shape of the wound. These dressings are usually dispensed in a sachet or tube. The second type of hydrogel is characterized by its fixed three-dimensional macro structure and it is usually presented as a flat sheet, e.g. Geliperm, Vigilon Spenco Second Skin or Clearsite (Figure 4.6).

Hydrogels have been described as 'tactile liars', due to their inaccurate sensation of feeling moist and cold [14].

At one time all hydrogels required a secondary dressing, but now there is a choice between those with or without a film protective layer.

The ability of hydrogel sheet dressings to reduce the sensation of pain and facilitate atraumatic removal makes them highly acceptable to the patient. Hydrogels have a key role to play in the management of flat and cavity wounds; however, care must be exercised if the wound is infected [15,16].

Hydrogel can be used successfully as a cavity filler.

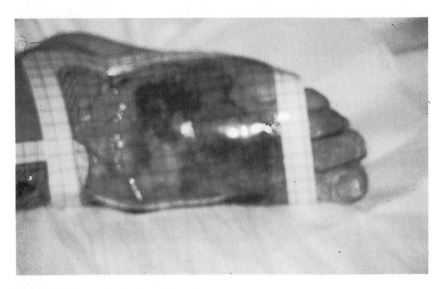

Figure 4.6 Clearsite hydrogel dressing.

HYDROCOLLOIDS

The introduction of the first hydrocolloid dressing by Convatec in the mid 1970s was based on successful management using Orbase for skin excoriation caused by effluent leaking from stomas and gastrointestinal fistulae.

Hydrocolloids (Figure 4.7) like Granuflex (Duoderm) and Granuflex E contain a number of constituents such as methycellulase (CMC), pectin, gelatin and a hydrophobic polymer. These constituents are based together to produce a gel forming matrix covered by an outer waterproof layer of polyurethane foam.

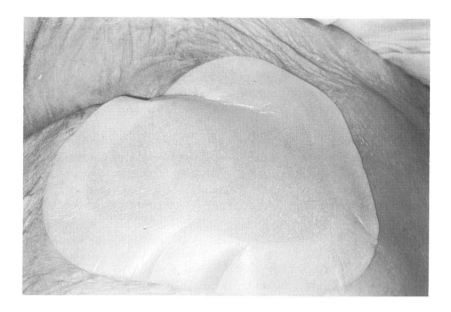

Figure 4.7 Granuflex hydrocolloid dressing.

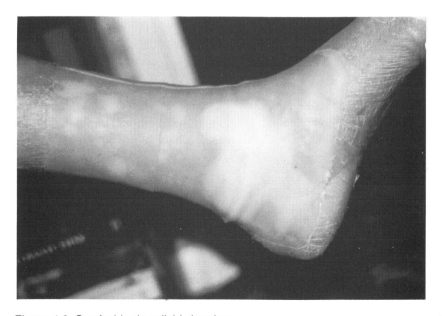

Figure 4.8 Comfeel hydrocolloid dressing.

Other hydrocolloid dressings include a range of products called Comfeel (Coloplast) which have a unique bevelled edge (Figure 4.8) whereas Tegasorb (3M) are oval shaped dressings in different sizes.

Hydrocolloid dressings are manufactured in a variety of thicknesses, e.g. Granuflex Extrathin/Comfeel Transparent, which enables clinical observation of the wound. Hydrocolloid paste, powder and granules are also available for use as cavity wound fillers or where wounds are more heavily exuding.

When a hydrocolloid dressing comes into contact with the wound exudate it interacts to produce a gel. Some gels, e.g. Granuflex, are known to produce an odour which has in the past been confused with the formation of pus. Ideally, hydrocolloid dressings are suitable for low to medium exuding wounds. They can also be used to successfully rehydrate and debride necrotic and sloughing tissue, alone or combined with enzyme or xerogels. Hydrocolloid dressings may be used in the presence of clinical infection (but not if the organism is aerobic) providing the patient is prescribed systemic antibiotics. They require no secondary dressing and the frequency of dressing change is determined by the amount of exudate. All manufacturers give clear guidance on any changes occurring in the outer dressing layer, combined with a swelling under the film which indicates when to change the dressing, or, as with the Comfeel pressure relieving dressing, when the foam discs are more than 50% thinner than their original size (Figure 4.9).

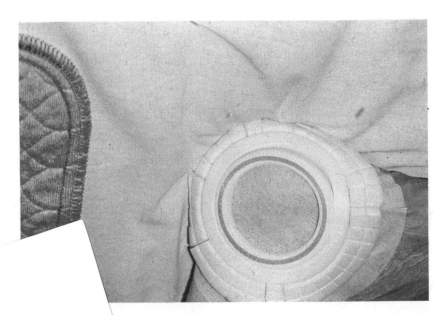

el pressure-relieving dressing.

The constituents of these dressings stimulate proliferation of granulation tissue and facilitate healing by providing a moist, warm environment complemented by a low adherent contact layer which enables trauma and pain-free removal. Hydrocolloid dressings also provide an intact barrier to micro-organisms [17].

A study [18] of the local environment of chronic wounds under Granuflex found the oxygen tension (PO_2) extremely low and the pH of the exudate more acidic. The combination of zero and low PO_2 allied with an increased acidity at the wound interface appeared to have a therapeutic effect by inhibiting the growth of bacteria, like pseudomonas. Studies have also revealed an increase in PO_2 of the wound tissues, as a result of enhanced wound angiogenesis [19] due to the artificially hypoxic state created under the dressing. A more recent study [20] also demonstrated increased fibrinolytic activity. Fibrin in the form of a fibrin cuff is frequently found wrapped around blood vessels of patients with varicose ulceration of the lower limbs or lipodermatosclerosis seriously disrupting perfusion and the diffusion of oxygen to the tissues. The tissues are subsequently compromised and necrosis may result. Clinical trials suggest that the wearing of a hydrocolloid dressing may help to reverse the situation by improving capillary function. Research findings indicate strong support for moist wound healing theory [21-3, 26].

XEROGELS

Xerogels are often referred to as polysaccharide beads, paste or granules. These dressings have evolved from the traditional use of honey and commercial dressings currently available include Debrisan (Pharmacia), Iodosorb/Iodoflex (Perstorp Pharma) and Dermaproof (Fermatec).

In practice Debrisan paste, consisting of spherical shaped beads of dextranomer, appears to be the easiest and most effective to use, although all forms are absorbent due to their hydrophilic abilities and can be used on wounds which are infected, contain pus, slough or other debris. As Debrisan is not biodegradable it must be removed. If the granules have been allowed to dry out they will adhere to the wound, necessitating rehydration and gentle irrigation to remove them. Some studies suggst that Debrisan may stimulate the formation of granulation tissues due to its fibrinolytic activity in improving the local capillary action.

The action of Debrisan can be enhanced by using a hydrocolloid or film dressing.

Iodosorb ointment, Iodosorb paste and Iodoflex (Perstorp Pharma) are three forms of cadexomer iodine (Figure 4.10). Iodosorb powder

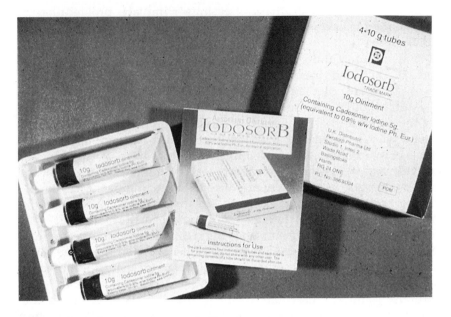

Figure 4.10 Iodosorb cadexomer iodine.

consists of hydrophilic beads containing 0.9% w/w iodine. The poly-saccharide chains are pushed apart as it absorbs moisture. The sterile powder is packaged in sachets and has the appearance of being yellow-brown in colour. In the presence of moisture 1 gm of Iodosorb is said to be able to absorb up to 7 ml of fluid [6]. As the beads swell the iodine is slowly liberated and transported by the capillary network at the wound interface. Excess wound exudate, plasma, pus and other wound debris are absorbed into the cadexomer gel and any bacteria, fungi or yeasts that pass into the gel are killed by the iodine. The action of the cadexomer dressing prevents the formation of fibrinogen involved in scab formation, so helping to facilitate epithelialization. A reduction of pain at the wound site can be attributed to the absorp-tion of prostaglandins. Odour is also reduced due to the eradication of odour producing bacteria. Cadexomer iodine is also available in the form of an ointment contained in a sterile tube. There are also two presentations of the product: a 6 × 4 cm (5 gm) and 8 × 6 cm (10 gm) dressing called Iodoflex. The cadexomer iodine paste is sandwiched between two pieces of gauze which are removed on application. A maximum of 50 gm of dressings can be used if the wound is larger. A single course of treatment should not continue for longer than three months.

A colour change is observed as the iodine is slowly utilized; when the dressing appears cream or white it should be renewed. Iodosorb and Iodoflex are biodegradable due to their sensitivity to enzymatic hydrolysis. Polysaccharide dressings are most suitable for slough and clinically infected wounds such as leg ulcers, pressure sores and some postsurgical complications. A secondary dressing of choice is required.

It is often difficult to determine an optimum time for changing the dressing as these products require a secondary dressing. However, as the product is biodegradable it is not necessary to remove all traces of it, as with Debrisan.

ODOUR ABSORBING DRESSINGS

There are several deodourizing dressings available containing activated charcoal to combat and reduce odour associated with clinical infection or fungating wounds. These include Kaltocarb (Britcair), Carbonet (Smith & Nephew), Actisorb Plus (Johnson & Johnson) and Lyofoam C (Ultra).

Practitioners will be familiar with malodorous wounds, particularly those caused by specific anaerobic organisms like the bacteroides or, less commonly, *Clostridium welchii*. Anaerobes tend to produce strong 'meaty type' odours wheras the aerobes such as klebsiella, proteus and pseudomonas spp. tend to produce strong 'fishy' odours. Necrotic areas or tissues that have been compromised are particularly prone to invasion by pathogenic organisms and the development of clinical infection.

Odour producing molecules are either drawn into the charcoal fabric of the dressing and trapped or, in the case of larger molecules, absorbed onto the wound contact layer.

Kaltocarb contains activated charcoal that has been bonded to a primary contact dressing of calcium alginate and backed with a layer of polyester viscose. The presence of the calcium alginate forms a moist healing environment and reduces odour.

Carbonet has a primary contact low adherent layer of Tricotex, an absorbent cotton viscose (Melolin fleece) layer covered with a fine polyethylene net next to the activated charcoal layer, followed by another layer of fine polyethylene net and polyester fleece. This dressing is less likely to absorb toxins and bacteria as the charcoal layer is not in direct contact with the wound [6].

Actisorb is 100% pure charcoal and contains silver which prevents bacterial growth on the actual dressing. This dressing can also help to reduce the excessive exudate frequently associated with malodorous wounds. Actisorb can be used on top of a low adherent dressing.

Lyofoam C has an activated charcoal layer which is sandwiched and sealed between a layer of Lyofoam and a thin layer of polyurethane foam. As exudate is absorbed horizontally across the hydrophobic dressing surface the charcoal remains dry and hence active against odour producing agents.

To date, very little valid clinical evidence exists on the comparative use of odour absorbing dressings, although their value in reducing and combating odour must be acknowledged and included in every wound product formulary. An alternative to the commercially manufactured dressings is the use of a thick or thin sugar paste, developed at Northwick Park Hospital. The absence of toxic effects on wounds treated with sugar paste may make it preferable to antiseptics for the management of dirty or infected wounds [25].

TOPICAL ANTIBIOTICS

As a general rule antibiotics should not be applied topically to wounds but given systemically [14], due to the risk of delayed healing from sensitivity reactions.

ANTIBACTERIALS

Products in this range include Flamazine (Smith & Nephew), metronidazole and Metrolop (Farmitalia Carlo Erba). Flamazine is a hydrophilic cream containing 1% silver sulphadiazine. This product is widely used to prevent the spread of Gram negative pathogenic organisms in patients with leg ulcers and burns, due to its broad spectrum antibacterial properties. Practitioners must avoid the product coming into contact with surrounding skin as maceration may occur. The necessity for frequent dressing changes, risk of leucopenia and the difficulty of maintaining an optimum environment for healing must be carefully considered.

Metronidazole has been shown to reduce odour and temporarily eradicate anaerobes when used topically. Researchers have observed that pathogenic organisms can re-emerge in the wound on cessation of the treatment. Prolonged use of these topical products is not desirable due to the possibility of inducing antibiotic resistance. Their value in treating fungating malodorous carcinomas is acknowledged.

The combination of metronidazole powder with a hydrogel is also effective in treating the odour associated with extensive tissue necrosis.

ANTISEPTICS

Although antiseptics are widely used and marginally preferable to antibiotics or antibacterial agents, their therapeutic value when used to irrigate a wound is debatable. Antiseptics used in this way have very little effect and if traditional solutions are used, these may have a toxic effect on healing tissues and delay the healing process. The controversy over chlorinated solutions has been reviewed [24].

Toxicity to fibroblasts, even at low concentrations of cetrimide containing products, has been noted [24]. Cleansing agents like hydrogen peroxide, when used on contaminated tissue, have their antiseptic effects reduced. The chemical reaction which is produced when the hydrogen peroxide reacts with catalase causes frothing, which helps to dislodge debris and slough. The report in the *Journal of the Medical Defence Union* on the death of a patient from an air embolism attributed to the use of hydrogen peroxide on a cavity wound highlights the need for caution [25].

Proflavine is often used in conjunction with ribbon gauze to pack a cavity wound. Clinical experience repeatedly shows that this type of dressing dries out in the wound even when changed twice daily. The released proflavine from the emulsion base is considered poor when in an aqueous based solution, hence diminishing its antimicrobial activity. Ribbon gauze packs can traumatize the wound due to their adherence when drying out. Some patients require strong analgesia prior to dressing change to reduce the pain experienced. More suitable alternatives are available which also facilitate wound healing, such as alginate cavity dressings, hydrogels and Allevyn cavity dressings.

The use of sterile water or sodium chloride is preferable in most instances as a cleansing solution. If antiseptics are required, then use should be clearly identified, duration defined and progress monitored.

DESLOUGHING AGENTS

Desloughing agents such as hyrocolloids, hydrogels and sugar paste have already been mentioned. Others include Aserbine (Bencard), a propylene glycol base containing malic, benzoic and salicylic acids, available as either a solution or cream. (The solution is six times more potent than the cream) and Malatese (Norton) solution. Both products require application at least twice daily. Enzyme preparations, like Varidase (Lederle), contain a mixture of streptokinase, a powerful proteolytic enzyme, and streptodornase which has nucleolytic properties. Together these enzymes produce an ideal biological wound cleanser. Clinical research indicates Varidase is a more effective cleanser than products like Betadine (povidone iodine) [27].

The removal of necrotic tissue and slough from a wound can be enhanced when Varidase is reconstituted with 5 ml of sterile water and combined with a hydrogel or inert gel (KY Jelly). Rehydration and separation of debris and dead tissues is facilitated if the wound is covered by a film or hydrocolloid dressing.

Practitioners should avoid shaking the reconstituted solution as the enzymes are easily denatured.

PASTE BANDAGES

There are five groups of medicated paste bandages currently available in the United Kingdom; most contain zinc oxide. All paste bandages require a secondary dressing and are designed to treat specific skin conditions associated with ulceration of the lower limbs, not the actual ulcer. For ease of reference the information has been produced in a table (see Table 6.9).

Despite the introduction of alternative methods of combating skin problems associated with ulceration, paste bandages are still widely used, especially in the community. Practitioners should familiarize themselves with the manufacturer's instructions on the use, application and removal of the bandages.

REFERENCES

1. United Kingdom Central Council (1984) *Code of Professional Conduct for Nurses, Midwives and Health Visitors*, UKCC, London.
2. Moody, M. (1993) Wound dressings. Principle of choice, part 1. RCN Nursing Update. *Nursing Standard*, 7, 9–14.
3. Turner, T.D. (1985) *Semiocclusive and Occlusive Dressing in an Environment for Healing: The Role of Occlusion*, International Congress and Symposium Series Number 88, (ed. T. Ryan), Royal Society of Medicine, London, pp. 5–14.
4. Winter, G.D. (1971) Healing of skin wounds and the influence of dressings on the repair process, in *Surgical Dressings and Wound Healing*, (ed. K.J. Harkiss), Crosby and Lockwood, London, pp. 46–60.
5. Fairbrother, J.E. (1988) Beyond occlusion and back again, in *Beyond Occlusion: Wound Care Proceedings*, International Congress and Symposium Series Number 136 (ed. T. Ryan), Royal Society of Medicine, London, pp. 3–8.
6. Thomas, S. (1990) *Wound Management and Dressings*, The Pharmaceutical Press, London.
7. Moody, M. (1992) Looking for non-adherence. *Nursing Times*, **88**(19), 65–8.
8. Thomas, S., Loveless, P. and Hay, N.P. (1988) Comparative review of the properties of six semipermeable film dressings. *Pharmaceut J*, **240**, 785–9.

9. Ritter, E.J. *et al.* (1987) Teratogenicity of di = (2-ethylhexyl) = phthalate, 2-ethylhexand, 2-ethylhexanoic acid and valproic acid and potentiation by caffeine. *Teratology*, **35**, 531–7.

10. Jarvis, S.P.M. *et al.* (1987) *How does Calcium Alginate Achieve Haemostasis in Surgery?* Paper presented to the International Congress on Thrombosis and Haemostasis, Brussels.

11. Moody, M.(1993) Evaluation of a semipermeable polyurethane absorptive dressing. *Prof Nurse*, **12**, 798–802.

12. Moody, M. (1991) Calcium alginate; a dressing trial. *Nursing Standard* (suppl.), **4,5**(50), 3–6.

13. Thomas, S. (1989) Pain in wound management. *Nursing Times* (suppl.), **88**, 11–15.

14. Morgan, D.A. (1994) *Formulary of Wound Management Products, A Guide for Health Care Staff*, 6th edn, obtainable from Media Medics Publications Ltd, 51 West Street, Chichester PO19 1RR.

15. Brennan, S.S. *et al.* (1983) *Infection and Healing under Hydrogel Occlusive Dressing is a Clear Advance in Wound Healing.* Proceedings of a Conference, Oxford, pp. 49–62.

16. Leaper, D.J. *et al.* (1984) Experimental infection and hydrogel dressings. *J Hosp Infection* (suppl.), **5**, 69–73.

17. Dunn, W. and Wilson, P. (1990) Evaluating the permeability of hydrocolloid dressings to multiresistant *Staphylococcus aureus*. *Pharmaceut J*, **245**, 248–50.

18. Vaghese, M.D. *et al.* (1986) Local environment of chronic wounds under synthetic dressings. *Arch Dermatol*, **122**, 52–7.

19. Cherry, G.W. and Ryan, T.J. (1985) *Enhanced Wound Angiogenesis with a new Hydrocolloid Dressing in an Environment for Healing: The Role of Occlusion*, International Congress and Symposium Series Number 88, (ed. T. Ryan), Royal Society of Medicine, London, 61–8.

20. Lydon, M.J. *et al.* (1988) Fibrinolytic activity of hydrocolloid dressings, in *Beyond Occlusion: Wound Care Proceedings*, International Congress and Symposium Series Number 136, (ed. T. Ryan), Royal Society of Medicine, London, 9–17.

21. Forrest, R.D. (1982) Early history of wound treatment. *J Roy Soc Med*, **75**, 198–205.

22. Hinman, C.C. (1963) Effects of air exposure and occlusion on experimental human skin wounds. *Nature*, **200**, 377–9.

23. Winter, G.D. (1962) Formation of scab and rate of epithelialization of superficial wounds in the skin of the young domestic pig. *Nature*, **193**, 293–4.

24. Morgan, D.A. (1991) Wound care, chlorinated solutions – an update. *J Tissue Viability*, **1**(2), 31–3.

25. Thomas, S. and Hay, N.P. (1985) Wound cleansing. *Pharmaceut J* (letter), 235–206.

26. Turner, T. (1985) Which dressing and why, in *Wound Care* (Ed. S. Westaby), Heinemann, London.

27. Graham-Brown, R.A.G. *et al.* (1983) A comparative study of the safety and efficiency of topical enzymatic therapy vs standard antiseptic dressings in the cleansing of leg ulcers. *Annales Chirugiae et Gynaecologicael*, **72**, 43–8.

Pressure sores 5

A pressure sore is an area of tissue necrosis (tissue death) due to excessive pressure for that individual, usually over a bony prominence. Barton theorized two processes (which commonly coexist) which cause reduced tissue perfusion of blood and its nutrients eventually resulting in anoxic (lack of oxygen) damage and necrosis [1]. The two processes are exclusion of blood from the skin of healthy individuals by the application of sustained pressure in excess of mean capillary pressure (this is 32 mmHg in young fit people) [2], and thrombosis of the microcirculation caused by disruptive and shearing forces. Thus pressure, friction, shear (and moisture) can be directly implicated in the damage caused to skin and the underlying subcutaneous tissues.

Numerous terms are used interchangeably in the literature such as decubitus ulcer, bedsore and pressure sore. Decubitus comes from the Latin *decumbere*, to lie down, alluding to the frequency of pressure sores in the immobile and bedridden. The term 'pressure sore' most accurately reflects the aetiology of the damage.

HISTORY

Pressure sores are not a 20th century occurrence – they have been around a very long time. When the embalmed body of an elderly Priestess of Amen (Egyptian XXI Dynasty) was examined by British Egyptologists in the British Museum at the turn of the century there was evidence of a large pressure sore over both the buttocks and shoulders [3]. In addition, in an effort to restore her body for her journey to the next world, her embalmers had used gazelle skin to cover the defects, a form of skin grafting. There are Biblical references [4] and pressure sores are mentioned in the writings of Moses Maimonides and Ambrose Paré [5, 6].

Four hundred years ago Fabricius suggested that pressure sores were caused by a 'pneum' resulting from nerve severance and loss of blood supply [7]. In 1749 Quesnay subclassified pressure sores into those caused by pressure and those due to other diseases [8]. By 1852 Brown-Sequard had concluded that skin pressure and moisture were the important aetiological factors, this view being supported by his work using paralysed animals and the fact that he could not produce ulcers if the skin was kept dry [9]. In 1873 Paget wrote 'Bedsores may be defined as the sloughing and mortification or death of a part produced by pressure' [10]. Medical interest virtually halted when in 1879 Charcot, the most prominent physician of his generation, produced his theory of causation [11]. In this he proposed that nerve injury released a neurotrophic factor leading to tissue necrosis. This factor could not be isolated using current techniques so pressure sores and, by implication, all wound care became the province of nurses, leaving doctors free to move onto the next conquerable heights. Compounding this pessimistic view was the work of Leyden claiming that sores were inevitable in desensitized skin [12].

So profound was the medical nihilism after Charcot's departure from the field that the ripples of disinterest reached as far as archaeology. The national wave of fervour for all things Egyptian was at its peak when the Priestess of Amen was being unwrapped and examined. In the British Museum's Egyptology department are vast tomes detailing the medical curiosities found during examination – kidney stones, foetuses, operation marks, etc. – yet the discovery of pressure sores and their subsequent grafting receives but a few words, an indication of their perceived unimportance. Some voices were trying to be heard during this time, with van Gehuchten in 1908 discussing the causal factors of muscle wasting and atony and Kuster drawing attention to the role of bacterial infection [13, 14]. In 1914, Marie and Roussy asserted that not only paraplegics but also debilitated patients developed pressure sores and, more importantly, that both prevention and treatment were feasible.

The second historical era and indeed renaissance of the subject occurred with World War 2. Large numbers of young paraplegics and debilitated people developed pressure sores and their surgical treatment began with the work of Davis [15], who suggested the use of pedicle flaps to treat ulceration, and Scoville and later Lamon and Alexander who reported the first successful use of excision and primary closure of sacral sores in patients protected by parenteral penicillin [16, 17]. Since then numerous authors have described various surgical techniques such as rotation flaps, skin grafts, 'S' flaps, etc. The removal of bony prominences has also been advocated to enhance surgical success rates.

We are now in the era of therapeutic intervention and the holistic approach to wound care. There are numerous important themes which are expanded upon in this or other chapters. They include the role of moist wound healing, possibly one of the greatest advances in our knowledge base concerning wound care [18]. This theme continues into the use and evaluation of wound dressings and the era of hydrocolloids, hydrogels, alginates, semipermeable membranes and interactive dressings. As we understand more about causation (pathophysiology) we correspondingly learn more about prevention and management. This has implications in the fields of biomechanics and the development of patient support systems as well as the role of risk assessment scores and prevention protocols. Scientific research can be at the forefront of patient care with tissue oxygenation, pressure loading, shear forces and temperature/moisture levels all being studied. The promotion and indeed enhancement of tissue repair and the role of growth factors are areas set to be at the head of molecular biology research into the next century.

PATHOPHYSIOLOGY

It is now accepted that pressure per se is one of the main causes of pressure sore formation [19–23]. Pressure that overcomes the capillary closure average of 32 mmHg will cause skin death, especially over a bony prominence [24]. There is ongoing debate as to what may constitute capillary closure pressures in the old and frail or the very sick [25]. Tissue anoxia and cell death lead to a process of inflammation[26]. Early relief from such pressure can reverse this trend (active hyperaemia is due to the vasodilatation response to injury) [27]. Irreversible damage has been shown to occur with pressures around 70 mmHg after two hours [28] and clinically we have all seen it occur faster than that in very ill patients. Bony prominences generate the highest pressures over the bone deep in the tissues. A clinically important finding and presumably a physiological adaptation is that relieving pressure for as little as five minutes allows the tissue to withstand higher pressures for longer [29]. Barton's work highlights the role of friction and shear[1].

Causes of pressure sores can usefully be divided into extrinsic (those which affect the type and degree of external pressure applied) and intrinsic (the physical states which put people at special risk) and are listed in Tables 5.1 and 5.2.

The common sites for pressure sore development include the sacrum, ischial tuberosities (what we sit on), hips, heels, elbows and, less commonly, knees, ankles and occiput. The majority occur over the sacrum, the area exposed to the full weight of a reclining person. Shocked and dehydrated patients after a femoral neck fracture can spend 12 hours lying on unprotected trolleys in Accident and

Table 5.1 Extrinsic causes

- Application of pressure/friction/shearing forces
- Moistened/macerated skin

Table 5.2 Intrinsic causes

- Biological age (may differ from chronological age)
- Neurological disease, e.g. paraplegia, peripheral neuropathy, stroke, Parkinson's disease, multiple sclerosis, Alzheimer's disease, etc.
- Cardiovascular disease
- Nutrition and body mass (build)
- Drugs
- Pain
- Incontinence
- Conscious level/ability to move
- Acute illness

Emergency departments [30]. Standard hospital mattresses have a shorter working life and produce higher pressures than Vaperm mattresses yet they are still in common use [31]. Pressure sores can be induced by poor mattress covers, poor lifting techniques inducing shear and friction and by tucking the feet in (heels are vulnerable due to the junction of two skin types). Nursing sick people in chairs can cause sores over the ischial tuberosities [32, 33] indicating that there is very little place for this practice.

Elderly people are one of the most at-risk groups in the population. They tend to suffer disproportionately from neurological and cardiovascular disease and more frequent hospital admissions. Sick elderly people are at great risk of developing pressure sores, acute illness being the single most important factor. Sedatives and excessive analgesia reduce pressure-pain sensation, decrease body movements and can cause hypotension (low blood pressure), dehydration and constipation. Patients in severe pain may need effective regular analgesia to allow them to cooperate with pressure relieving therapy and rehabilitation. Double incontinence is highly associated with pressure sore formation, an extrinsic effect and an indication of severe illness. In elderly people the presentation of acute illness is often non-specific (falls, incontinence, confusion and immobility) and may be missed until pressure sore damage occurs.

Common factors preceding the development of pressure sores in elderly people include an acute illness, an injury or fall, anaesthetic or operation, acute confusional state, dehydration, constipation (aetiology unknown though high rectal pressures are one theory), sedation and a change of environment.

SKIN BLOOD FLOW AND CUTANEOUS OXYGEN

In 1851 von Gerlach studied the diffusion of oxygen through human skin [34]. The measurement of arterial PO_2 via skin was pioneered by Baumberger in 1951 and further developed by Roth [35, 36]. By 1969 Huch was using nicotinic acid to vasodilate the skin on the scalp of newborn infants to measure their PO_2 and showed that it equated well to arterial oxygen [37]. The next technical advance was the use of heated sensors [38] and Bader has developed this technique to look at changes in transcutaneous oxygen with the application and relief of pressure and has identified the recovery characteristics of soft tissues after the relief of pressure with graphs of transcutaneous oxygen [39,40]. It is now possible to measure transcutaneous oxygen and carbon dioxide though the role of CO_2 is obscure. This type of measurement is at the forefront of one aspect of research into pressure sores.

MANAGEMENT AND PREVENTION

Preventing pressure sores requires an understanding of their causation, a knowledge of those groups of people most at risk and the application of those two components to a prevention plan. The majority of pressure sores are preventable and hence the onus is on the medical and nursing professions to accept this responsibility. Hitherto pressure sores have been seen as purely the nurses' domain and hence their problem. This can no longer be justified. Total care of patients is a multidisciplinary process and the role of doctors in prevention and management is crucial.

Skin integrity should be seen as one of the vital components of the peripheral circulation. As such it must be considered at the very outset of medical intervention. This means that tissue integrity in its widest sense must form part of the doctor's immediate assessment and intervention arranged urgently in the form of support aids if required. If this is done the more detailed assessment can take place without further damage occurring. Failure at this stage or at later stages to assess and determine risk (especially with intercurrent illnesses or a worsening of a condition) lays the whole team open to litigation. There are few specialties without patients at risk in a hospital setting and developing plans to look after more frail and ill people at home means that these same issues will confront community teams.

The key principles of pressure sore management are outlined below:

- Bedrest – on suitable support system, e.g., APAM
- Nutrition – repeated assessments of hydration and nutrition (see Chapter 2)
- Pain relief – may need opiate preparations
- Anti-inflammatory and immunosuppressive drugs – try and stop if possible

- Antibiotics – treat cellulitis with parenteral antibiotics, never topically
- Debridement – contentious, wounds debride naturally if pressure is relieved
- Antiseptics – clean wounds with saline, avoid antiseptics
- Dressings – see Chapter 4
- Plastic surgery – in appropriate patients cavity wounds should have a plastic surgery opinion early in the management planning

PREVENTION

Predicting risk

A classic study in 1975 found that elderly patients admitted to hospital were at very high risk of developing pressure sores [40]. From this study was developed the Norton pressure sore prediction score using five patient features: physical condition, mental state, activity, mobility and incontinence. It has been subsequently joined by a plethora of other scores including the Waterlow [42] (Figures 5.1 and 5.2) and in the US the Braden scale [43]. This has been extensively evaluated amongst nurses and does well in these critical evaluations.

Using risk assessment scales to predict pressure sore problems is only one aspect of the prevention plan. The timing of their use and repeat assessments, especially at times of acute illness, all have to be considered. They are an aid, not a substitute for good management and prevention.

General measures

The largest at-risk group of people will be the ill elderly. This usually means at least a period of bedrest and close attention paid to food and fluid intake and bowel and bladder needs. Seriously ill or already dehydrated people will require intravenous fluids. Nutritional requirements should be assessed early so that a decision can later be made concerning either parenteral feeding (via an intravenous line), supplements or total feeding via a finebore nasogastric tube or simple supplements orally. Protracted urinary incontinence may necessitate the use of a catheter in female patients though in some men a penile sheath may mean that a catheter is not required. Constipation must be treated early and faecal impaction avoided. If impaction is already present it should be treated with gentle manual removal and then the use of suppositories, **not** oral laxatives, especially stimulant ones like senna.

The skin over at-risk sites should be kept clean and dry. Harsh soaps and cleansing agents must be avoided (they cause excessive dryness and irritation). There is no good evidence that massage helps prevent

REMEMBER: TISSUE DAMAGE OFTEN STARTS PRIOR TO ADMISSION, IN CASUALTY. A SEATED PATIENT IS ALSO AT RISK

ASSESSMENT: (See over) IF THE PATIENT FALLS INTO ANY OF THE RISK CATEGORIES THEN PREVENTATIVE NURSING IS REQUIRED.
A COMBINATION OF GOOD NURSING TECHNIQUES AND PREVENTATIVE AIDS WILL DEFINITELY BE NECESSARY.

PREVENTION:

PREVENTATIVE AIDS:

Special Mattress/Bed:
- 10 + Overlays or specialist foam mattresses
- 15 + Alternating pressure overlays, mattresses bed systems
- 20 + Bed Systems: Fluidised, bead, low air loss and alternating pressure mattresses.

Note: Preventative aids cover a wide spectrum of specialist features. Efficacy in the 20+ area should be judged on the basis of independent evidence.

Cushions:
- No patient should sit in a wheelchair without some form of cushioning. If nothing else is available - use the patient's own pillow.
- 10 + 4" Foam cushion.
- 15 + Specialist Gel and/or foam cushion
- 20 + Cushion capable of adjustment to suit individual patient.

Bed Clothing:
- Avoid plastic draw sheets, inco pads and tightly tucked in sheets/sheet covers, especially when using Specialist bed and mattress overlay systems.
- Duvet - plus vapour permeable cover

NURSING CARE:

General:
- Frequent changes of position, lying or sitting.
- Use of pillows?

Pain
- Appropriate pain control

Nutrition
- High Protein, vitamins, minerals

Patient Handling:
- Correct lifting technique
- Hoists
- Monkey Pole
- Transfer devices

Patient Comfort Aids:
- Real sheepskins
- Bed cradle
- 4" cover plus adequate protection

Operating Table/
Theatre/A&E Trolley

Skin Care:
- General Hygiene, NO rubbing.
- Correct lifting and positioning.
- Cover with an appropriate dressing

IF TREATMENT IS REQUIRED, FIRST REMOVE PRESSURE

WOUND CLASSIFICATION

BLANCHING HYPERAEMIA	STAGE I	Is wound RED?	YES	Semi-permeable film hydrocolloid sheet
			NO	
NON-BLANCHING HYPERAEMIA	STAGE II	Is wound Red, clean but not healed?	YES	Hydrocolloid, alginate, hydrogel, Silastic Foam (deep)
			NO	
ULCERATION PROGRESSES	STAGE III	Is wound YELLOW/ infected/inflamed?	YES	Alginate, hydrogel, hydrocolloid
ULCERATION EXTENDS	STAGE IV	Infected?	YES	Alginate ribbon or rope, non adherent topical antimicrobial dressing, polysaccharide paste
			NO	
INFECTIVE NECROSIS	STAGE V	Is wound BLACK/ Necrotic?	YES	Debride-surgical excision, hydrocolloid, hydrogel, enzymatic treatment.
			NO	

Figure 5.1 Waterlow pressure sore prediction score. Reproduced with kind permission of Judy Waterlow.

WATERLOW PRESSURE SORE PREVENTION TREATMENT POLICY

RING SCORES IN TABLE, ADD TOTAL.   SEVERAL SCORES PER CATEGORY CAN BE USED

BUILD/WEIGHT FOR HEIGHT ★		SKIN TYPE VISUAL RISK AREAS ★		SEX AGE ★		SPECIAL RISKS ★	
AVERAGE	0	HEALTHY	0	MALE	1	TISSUE MALNUTRITION ★	
ABOVE AVERAGE	1	TISSUE PAPER	1	FEMALE	2	e.g.: TERMINAL CACHEXIA	8
OBESE	2	DRY	1	14–49	1	CARDIAC FAILURE	5
BELOW AVERAGE	3	OEDEMATOUS	1	50–64	2	PERIPHERAL VASCULAR	
		CLAMMY (TEMP↑)	1	65–74	3	DISEASE	5
		DISCOLOURED	2	75–80	4	ANAEMIA	2
		BROKEN/SPOT	3	81+	5	SMOKING	1

CONTINENCE ★		MOBILITY ★		APPETITE ★		NEUROLOGICAL DEFICIT ★	
COMPLETE/CATHETERISED	0	FULLY	0	AVERAGE	0	e.g.: DIABETES, M.S, CVA,	
OCCASION INCONT	1	RESTLESS/FIDGETY	1	POOR	1	MOTOR/SENSORY	
CATH/INCONTINENT OF FAECES	2	APATHETIC	2	N.G. TUBE/		PARAPLEGIA	4–6
DOUBLY INCONT	3	RESTRICTED	3	FLUIDS ONLY	2		
		INERT/TRACTION	4	NBM/ANOREXIC	3		
		CHAIRBOUND	5				

MAJOR SURGERY/TRAUMA ★		MEDICATION ★	
ORTHOPAEDIC BELOW WAIST, SPINAL	5	CYTOTOXICS	
ON TABLE >2 HOURS	5	HIGH DOSE STEROIDS	
		ANTI-INFLAMMATORY	4

SCORE	10+ AT RISK	15+ HIGH RISK	20+ VERY HIGH RISK

Figure 5.2 Waterlow pressure sore prevention/treatment policy. Reproduced with kind permission of Judy Waterlow.

pressure sores and some that it is positively harmful [44]. Barrier creams have a role when there is unavoidable wetness [44] but skin sensitization can occur.

People with sensory loss, e.g. paraplegics, usually do not feel any discomfort, hence the danger. Other at-risk people may feel uncomfortable but be unable to change position, e.g. severe arthritis, Parkinson's disease or simple weakness. Correct positioning for comfort and the changing of that position for the same reason are obviously vital. The use of two-hourly turns is a contentious issue. Frequent turning does help prevent pressure sores but the exact frequency of such turning is not known with any accuracy. A very ill frail elderly person may need turning hourly to be sure of adequate protection and this is rarely feasible or achievable. If it continues throughout the night as well (and for continued protection it should) then the patient may get very little rest. Staffing levels do not usually allow this form of prevention except in special circumstances. Someone at this much risk should be nursed on one of the support surfaces that does not require routine turning of the patient. Turning must still occur, however, for patient comfort on request.

There is no place in the care of patients for the routine use of restraints. Cot sides and fixed chair tables are dangerous and their use is not acceptable. Tilt-back chairs and fixed tray chairs should never be seen. A few people use a form of cot side at home, especially stroke patients, and hence their use in this specific way may be justified. Cot sides are dangerous, result in even more physical trauma to the patient than if they had fallen out of bed and are implicated with other restraints in pressure sore formation [46]. A very agitated patient needs skilled assessment and the cause found for the agitation. Treatment may not result in immediate subsidence of the problem and if falling out of bed is likely then the patient should be nursed on a mattress on the floor. The person's relatives need to have this method of management explained and the dignity and privacy of the confused or agitated person considered.

The concept that 'bed is bad' specially for older people has resulted in the pendulum swinging in favour of chair nursing. In the majority of cases this is a mistake. Pressure sores occur from sitting in chairs as the same issue of mobility and risk still apply [47]. Pressure is more effectively relieved in bed.

During the early stages of rehabilitation the person should be up for meals and commode/toilet only and for no longer than 15–30 minutes unless on a specialized alternating support. Treatment and activity via physiotherapy should if possible be carried out from bed to standing/walking and then back to bed. Unlimited chair sitting should only occur once the patient can move themselves into a comfortable position and even then most people recovering from a serious illness or who are extremely old and frail benefit from periods of rest on the bed.

Heel protection

Heels are at especial risk of pressure sore development. This is due to the junction of the two skin types occurring there, the thin sensitive skin over the back of the Achilles meeting the thick hard plantar skin of the heel proper, used to stand and weight bear. It is a very common site for pressure damage, as most of us can testify – a new pair of shoes exposes this weak area in a matter of minutes with blister formation from the pressure and friction/shear forces! Heels must be protected in all at-risk individuals. It may be sufficient to use such aids as a sheepskin fleece or bootee or to lift the heels off the mattress by the use of a pillow. In all cases the weight of the bedclothes must be removed by a bed cradle. High-risk individuals need an appropriate support system.

Pressure relieving mattresses

The majority of people will only need some form of pressure relieving mattress for a short period of time. Any such mattress, however, should be simple and easy to use, fairly portable and reliable. They should also be comparatively inexpensive. Highly specialized bulky and complicated support systems are invariably expensive and their use should be restricted to the comparatively few patients that need them. Pressure relieving mattresses fall into two subgroups: static low pressure (Table 5.3) and alternating pressure mattresses.

Table 5.3 Static low pressure mattresses

• Soft overlays
• Low pressure bed mattresses
• Air mattresses
• Flotation water beds
• Flotation air beds

Alternating pressure air mattresses – APAMs

A comprehensive description of the numerous types of support mattress has been provided by Bliss [48].

Soft overlays are very helpful in achieving comfort and do distribute some of the surface pressure. They are useful, therefore, in low-risk patients and to help relieve discomfort but they cannot be used to prevent pressure sores, especially those due to deep tissue pressure in the high-risk patient.

The low pressure bed mattresses have similar properties to the overlays. They are a distinct improvement on the standard NHS mattress and, either alone or together with soft overlays, are suited to the low-risk patient. The first water bed was designed by Arnott in the 1830s and one was reported in the *Lancet* in 1851 [49, 50]. Paget described both a water bed and a water mattress in his classic lecture presented at St Bartholomew's Hospital in 1873 [10]. The modern equivalents still have the same drawbacks. They are bulky, extremely heavy when full of water, need temperature regulation and make the management of the patient more difficult. The patient literally floats and hence eating, drinking and excreting can be fraught with wavelike movement resulting in seasickness. Rehabilitation is similarly restricted. They can have a specialized role in the care of immobile patients with distinct palliative care needs such as pain on movement, etc.

Flotation air beds similarly have some specialized uses, e.g. some burns patients, but do not have a role in the routine prevention or treatment of pressure sores.

No patient should be denied a specialized system on the grounds of cost but conversely an individual case must be made for why such a system is the correct one.

Alternating pressure air mattresses work on the principle of reproducing the body's own pressure defence mechanism, movement. In this way skin is exposed to higher than capillary closure pressures especially over bony surfaces but this pressure is then regularly relieved, allowing blood flow into the area and the occurrence of reactive hyperaemia. There are various makes and types of APAM ranging from the simple to the sophisticated. The simple APAMs are effective but can be unreliable (detachment of air tubes, motor malfunction). The horizontal cells must be greater than 10 cm in diameter to be effective. Most APAMs work on a 7–10 minute deflation/reflation cycle and some offer complex waveforms of movement through various layers. All appear to be equally effective but reliability often determines choice.

APAMs are the support system of choice for the routine prevention of pressure sores in medium to high-risk patients. They should be in place under the patient as soon after contact with the health professionals (hospital and community) as is practicable. This means they should be available in ambulances and A & E departments, X-ray, etc. as well as in the boot of the car when a community nurse or GP visits a likely candidate who will probably remain at home. The person may only need the APAM for a few days and then be well enough to transfer to a static support system, thus ensuring efficient use of resources. Any new worsening of a patient's condition, however, is an indication to return to the APAM.

Table 5.4 Alternating pressure air mattresses

- Ripple bed (large cell)
- Bubble pad
- Alphacare
- Nimbus mattress
- Pegasus airwave bed (Figure 5.1)

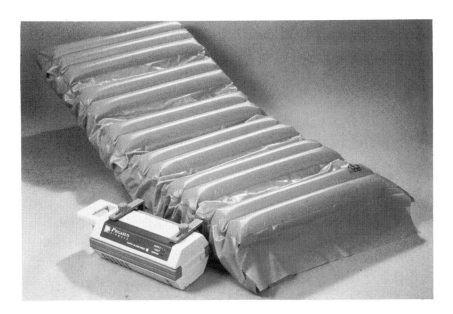

Figure 5.3 Example of an APAM.

Special considerations

At home a bed may be softer and the provision of a bed cradle and heel protection may be sufficient in a mild illness. Nursing a very sick person at home will require planning for all the continence requirements, nutrition and bed protection as well as the provision of an APAM. Duvets are much lighter and not prone to be tucked in, trapping heels. Drawsheets and sheets should not be of coarse linen and should be checked regularly to ensure they have not become wrinkled and hence are cutting into the skin.

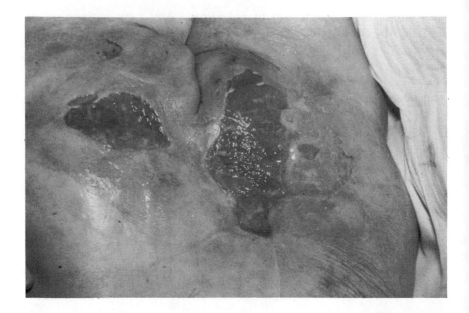

Figure 5.4 Pressure sore - superficial.

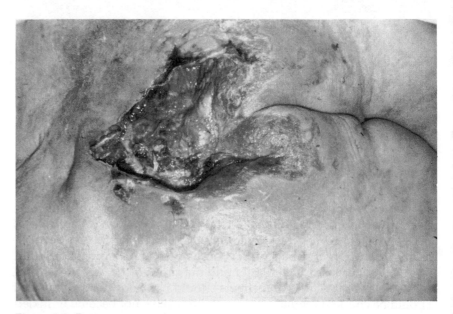

Figure 5.5 Pressure sore - deep.

At home people do sometimes die; in hospital they have a cardiac arrest! The resuscitation status of every hospital patient should be known to the health care professionals concerned and if a cardiac arrest situation is likely an APAM should be used that can be collapsed immediately. APAM chair and wheelchair cushions are currently being developed. Their use forms part of the expert assessment by occupational therapists and they have detailed knowledge of the other static cushion devices available. All need regular and expert maintenance.

Most pressure sores are preventable, even those of the terminally ill patient. Pressure area relief and the use of the most suitable support surface should be part of the holistic approach to palliative care. Palliative care may continue for a long period of time at home or in hospital and the avoidance or early treatment of pressure sores saves the person a further distressing complaint.

PRESSURE SORES (CLASSIFICATION)

The diagnosis of a pressure sore is part of the routine clinical practice of both nurses and doctors and many other health care workers can recognize them. There is marked disagreement, however, as to the various stages of tissue damage. Grading the severity of a pressure sore has been a subjective matter of clinical judgement and the wide variety of classifications has not brought uniformity of approach. The classifications range from the simple (Table 5.5) [51] to the more complicated (Table 5.6) [52].

Table 5.5 Classification of pressure sores

•	Grade 1	Discolouration of the skin
•	Grade 2	Superficial sore
•	Grade 3	Destruction of skin, no cavity
•	Grade 4	Destruction of skin, cavity

Table 5.6 Classification of pressure sores [53]

Stage 1
Blanching hyperaemia - momentary light finger pressure on to the site of erythema, following a prolonged period of pressure on the skin, causes the skin to blanch, indicating that the skin's microcirculation is intact.

Stage 2
Non-blanching erythema - the erythema remains when light finger pressure is applied, indicating some microcirculatory disruption. Superficial damage, including epidermal ulceration, may be present.

Stage 3
Ulceration progresses through the dermis to the interface with the subcutaneous tissue.

Table 5.6 *cont'd*

Stage 4

The ulcer extends into the subcutaneous fat. Underlying muscle is swollen and inflamed. The ulcer tends to spread laterally, temporarily impeded from downward progress by deep fascia.

Stage 5

Infective necrosis penetrates down to the deep fascia. Destruction of muscle now occurs rapidly.

Table 5.7 The U.K. consensus classification of pressure sore severity

---

The patient's pressure sore code is made up of four components and could look like this:

3.3.2.1

- The first number is the primary code: 1-4 graded for tissue involvement.
- The second number is the secondary code: 0-4 refinement of tissue involved.
- The third number is the nature of the wound bed: 0-4.
- The final number indicates infective complications: 0-2.

Each code has a corresponding clinical statement to allow accurate interpretation:

Stage 0   No clinical evidence of a pressure sore

0.0   Normal appearance, intact skin
0.1   Healed with scarring
0.2   Tissue damage, but not assessed as a pressure sore

Stage 1   Discolouration of intact skin – light finger pressure applied to the site does not alter the discolouration

1.1   Non-blanching erythema with increased local heat
1.2   Blue/purple/black discolouration

Stage 2   Partial thickness skin loss or damage involving epidermis and/or dermis

2.1   Blister
2.2   Abrasion
2.3   Shallow ulcer, without undermining of adjacent tissue
2.4   Any of these with underlying blue/purple/black discolouration or induration

Stage 3   Full thickness skin loss involving damage or necrosis of subcutaneous tissue but not extending to underlying bone, tendon or joint capsule

3.1   Crater, without undermining of adjacent tissue
3.2   Crater, with undermining of adjacent tissue
3.3   Sinus, the full extent of which is not certain
3.4   Full thickness skin loss but wound bed covered with necrotic tissue (hard or leathery black/brown tissue or softer yellow/cream/grey slough) which masks the true extent of the tissue damage. The ulcer is at least a Stage 3 sore. Until debrided it is not possible to observe whether damage extends into muscle or involves damage to bone or supporting structures

Table 5.7 *cont'd*

Stage 4 Full thickness skin loss with extensive destruction and tissue necrosis extending to underlying bone, tendon or joint capsule

4.1   Visible exposure of bone, tendon or joint capsule
4.2   Sinus assessed as extending to bone, tendon or joint capsule

Third digit classification for the nature of the wound bed

x.x0   Not applicable, intact skin
x.x1   Clean, with partial epithelialization
x.x2   Clean, with or without granulation, but no obvious epithelialization
x.x3   Soft slough, cream/yellow/green in colour
x.x4   Hard or leathery black/brown necrotic (dead/avascular) tissue

Fourth digit classification for infective complications

x.xx0   No inflammation surrounding the wound bed
x.xx1   Inflammation surrounding the wound bed
x.xx2   Cellulitis bacteriologically confirmed

This difficult state of affairs has been greatly helped by the work of Morison and Reid [53] who arranged a meeting of experts in the field to develop a classification of pressure sore severity that would be accepted nationally and internationally. This U.K. consensus classification (Table 5.7) will hopefully enable a true clinical consensus but also allow proper interpretation of the results of clinical trials in all aspects of pressure sore prevention and management.

REFERENCES

1.   Barton, A.A. and Barton, M. (1978) *The Management and Prevention of Pressure Sores*, Faber, London.
2.   Landis, E.M. (1930) Microinjection studies of capillary blood pressure in human skin. *Heart*, **15**, 209–28.
3.   Thompson, R.J. (1961) Pathological changes in mummies. *Proc R Soc Med*, 54, 409–15.
4.   *The Bible*, Isaiah 1:6.
5.   Maimonides, M. (1970) *The Medical Aphorisms of Moses Maimonides*, (trans. and ed. R.F. Bloch), Bloch Publishing for Yershia University Press, New York.
6.   Levine, J.M. (1992) Historical notes on pressure ulcers: the cures of Ambrose Paré. *Decubitus*, **2**, 23–6.
7.   Fabricius, H. (1593) *De gangrene et sphacelo tractatus methodicus*, 10th edn, J.T. de Bry, Leyden.
8.   Quesnay, M. (1749) *Traite de gangrene*, Paris, pp. 319–53.
9.   Brown-Sequard, E. (1853) *Experimental Researches Applied to Physiology and Pathology*, H. Baillière, New York.

10. Paget, J. (1873) Clinical lecture on bedsores. *Students J Hosp Gaz London*, **1**, 144.
11. Charcot, J.M. (1879) *Lectures on the Diseases of the Nervous System. Delivered at La Saltpetriere*, (trans. from 2nd edn by G. Sigerson), Henry C. Lea, Philadelphia.
12. Leyden, E. (1874) *Klinik de Ruckenmarks – Kraukheiten, vol. 1*, A. Hirchwald, Berlin, p. 156.
13. Van Gehuchten, A. (1908) *Neuraxe*, **10**, 298.
14. Kluster, I. (1908) Decubitus eulenberg. *Real Encyclopodie*, **3**, 671.
15. Davis, J.S. (1938) Operative treatment of scars following bedsores. *Surgery*, **3**, 1.
16. Scoville, W.B. (1967) Cited by Bailey, B.N. in *Bedsores*, Edward Arnold, London.
17. Lamon, J.C. and Alexander, E. (1945) Secondary closure of decubitus ulcers with the aid of penicillin. *JAMA*, **127**, 396.
18. Winter, B.D. (1962) Moist wound healing. *Nature*, **193**, 293–4.
19. Walden, R.H. *et al*. (1971) Inoperable pressure sores. Prevention and management. *NY State J Med*, **71**, 657.
20. Guttman, L. (1955) The problem of treatment of pressure sores in spinal paraplegics. *Br J Plast Surg*, **8**, 196.
21. Kosiak, M. *et al*. (1958) Evaluation of pressure as a factor in the production of ischial ulcers. *Arch Phys Med Rehab*, **39**, 623.
22. Exton-Smith, A.N. and Sherwin, R.W. (1961) The prevention of pressure sores – the significance of spontaneous bodily movement. *Lancet*, **ii**, 1124–6.
23. Reswick, J.B. and Simoes, N. (1975) Application of engineering principles in the management of spinal cord injured patients. *Clin Orthop*, **112**, 124.
24. Kosiak, M. (1959) Etiology and pathology of decubitus ulcers. *Arch Phys Med*, **40**, 62.
25. Rithalia, S.V.S. (1989) Comparison of pressure distribution in wheelchair seat cushions. *Care Sci Pract*, **7**(4), 87–9.
26. Kosiak, M. (1961) Etiology of decubitus ulcers. *Arch Phys Med*, **42**, 19.
27. Lewis, T. and Gant, R.T. (1825) Observations upon reactive hyperaemia in man. *Heart*, **12**, 73.
28. Kosiak, M. (1961) Etiology of decubitus ulcers. *Rehabil Rec*, **2**, 829.
29. Hussain, T. (1953) An experimental study of some pressure effects on tissue with reference to the bedsore problem. *J. Pathol Bacteriol*, **66**, 347.
30. Versluysen, M. (1986) How elderly patients with femoral fracture develop pressure sores in hospital. *Br Med J*, **292**, 1311–13.
31. Blenkinsop, G.K. (1988) An evaluation of the Vaperm mattress: Salisbury Health Authority 1985–1986. *Care Sci Pract*, **6**(3), 81–5.
32. David, J. (1981) The size of the problem of pressure sores. *Care Sci Pract*, **1**(1), 10–13.
33. Nyquist, R. and Hawthorn, P.J. (1987) The prevalence of pressure sores within an area health authority. *Nursing*, **12**, 183–7.
34. Von Gerlach, A. (1851) Uber das Hautatmen. *Arch Anat Physiol*, **431**, 479.
35. Baumberger, J. and Goodfriend, R. (1951) Determination of arterial oxygen tension in man by equilibration through intact skin. *Fed Proc Fed Am Socs Exp Biol*, 10, 10–11.

36. Roth, G., Sjostedt, S. and Caligara, F. (1957) Bloodless determination of arterial oxygen tension by polarography. *Science Tools LKW Instruments J*, **4**, 37–45.

37. Huch, A., Huch, R. and Lubbers, D. (1969) Quantative polarographische Sauertsoffdruck Messung auf der Kopfhaut des Neugeborenen. *Arch Gynaek*, **207**, 443–51.

38. Eberhard, P. *et al.* (1972) *Perkutane Messung des Sauerstoffpartialdrukkes Methodik und Anwendengen.* Proceedings of 'Medizin-Technik 1972', Stuttgart, p. 26.

39. Bader, D.L. and Gent, C.A. (1988) Changes in transcutaneous oxygen tension as a result of prolonged pressure at the sacrum. *Clin Physiol Meas*, **9**(1), 33–40.

40. Bader, D.L. (1990) The recovery characteristics of soft tissues following repeated loading. *J Rehab Res Dev*, **27**(2), 141–50.

41. Norton, D., McLaren, R. and Exton-Smith, A.N. (1975) *An Investigation of Geriatric Nursing Problems in Hospital*, Churchill Livingstone, Edinburgh.

42. Waterlow, J. (1988) The Waterlow card for the prevention and management of pressure sores: towards a pocket policy. *Care Sci Pract*, **6**(1), 8–12.

43. Braden, B.J. and Bergstrom, N. (1989) Clinical utility of the Braden scale for predicting pressure sore risk. *Decubitus*, **2**, 44–51.

44. Olson, B. (1990) Effects of massage for prevention of pressure ulcers. *Decubitus*, **2**, 32–7.

45. Hibbs, P.J. (1988) *Pressure Area Care for the City and Hackney Health Authority*, City and Hackney Health Authority, London.

46. Lofgren, R.P., Macpherson, D.S, Granieri, R. *et al.* (1989) Mechanical restraints on the medical wards: are protective devices safe? *Am J Public Health*, **79**, 735–8.

47. Lowthian, P.T. (1977) A review of pressure sores prophylaxis. *Nursing Mirror* (suppl.), **141**(2), 7–15.

48. Bliss, M.R. (1992) Pressure sore management and prevention, in *Textbook of Geriatric Medicine and Gerontology*, 4th edn, (eds J.C. Brocklehurst, R.C. Tallis and H.M. Fillit), Churchill Livingstone, Edinburgh.

49. Arnott, N. (1838) *Elements of Physics or Natural Philosophy, General and Medical, Vol. 1*, Lea and Blanchard, Philadelphia, pp. 499–507.

50. Anon. (1851) New inventions in aid of the practice of medicine and surgery. Water and air cushions and mattresses. *Lancet*, **1**(96).

51. Jordan, M. and Clark, M.O. (1977) *Report on the Incidence of Pressure Sores in the Patient Community of the Greater Glasgow Health Board Area on 21st January 1976.* University of Strathclyde, Glasgow.

52. Morison, M.J. (1990) *Pressure Sore Blueprint: Aetiology, Prevention and Management*, Conva Tec (UK), Uxbridge.

53. Reid, J. and Morison, M. (1994) Towards a consensus: classification of pressure sores. *J Wound Care*, **3**, 157–60.

Leg ulcers 6

One of the earliest known references to venous disorders of the lower limbs can be found in the papyrus of Ebers dated 1550 BC [1]. It would appear that there has been a considerable empirical understanding of the treatment of venous problems for at least 2000 years [2]. Despite all of this available knowledge leg ulcers represent an increasing drain on our national health care resources with approximately 2% of the budget being spent on venous disorders [3]. If current demographic trends continue as predicted for the elderly we shall have a 43% increase in people over the age of 85 by the year 2000 [4] and expenditure on treating leg ulcers will escalate significantly due to their high incidence in this very susceptible age group. Current treatment costs have been estimated in the range of £150–650 million per annum [5] but these figures have been disputed by Bosanquet [6] who suggests a figure of £230–400 million as more realistic. He based his calculation on treatment frequencies at Riverside (London (1990–91) and other local surveys adjusted to national rates through estimation of prevalence. As many as 50% of patients with leg ulcers still require treatment after one year [7] and many of those need three or more dressing changes per week [8], hence the conservative estimate of £1200 per patient per annum based on one visit per week by a district nurse may be considered as greatly underestimated.

A report by the Office of Health Economics in 1992 [3] indicated that £180 million was spent on time given by district nurses to treat leg ulcers, excluding any dressing products or support garments. General practitioner costs attributed to treating venous diseases of the legs were estimated at £8 million with an additional £7 million spent on prescriptions and a further £10 million on elastic hosiery (excluding compression bandages). Hospital inpatient costs for treating venous diseases total some £89 million.

Although there now exists much more awareness of costs in terms of treatment of venous ulcers, very little is known about costs in terms of reduced quality of life for the patient with a leg ulcer [9]. Hence it is difficult to quantify given the dearth of published information. As many patients (50%) have been shown to have a history of leg ulceration for ten or more years [10, 11], the need to understand the impact of venous ulceration on the quality of the patient's life is of paramount importance if an effective programme is to be developed and implemented. Hence the importance of addressing quality of life issues as outcome measures when auditing leg ulcer care [12]. Negative outcomes associated with the presence of peripheral vascular disease include limitation on physical mobility, low levels of energy, sleep disturbance, pain, emotional problems and social isolation [9].

EPIDEMIOLOGY

The precise incidence of leg ulceration remains unknown. This is partially due to the dearth of epidemiological studies and the lack of uniform diagnosis criteria since different types of vascular insufficiency problems often occur together in varying degrees and in various combinations [13].

A review of ten epidemiological studies [14] concluded that all had some limitations either in terms of population surveyed, techniques used to identify patients with venous disease and/or leg ulceration, the definitions used for prevalence of leg ulceration or size of sample assessed [14].

Studies [8, 15] estimate the prevalence of active leg ulcers in the United Kingdom to be between 0.15% and 0.18% of the total population, which equates to 100 000 people at any given time having one or more active leg ulcers. A further 300 000 people are acknowledged to be at risk of ulceration. Although the majority of people who present with ulceration of the leg are elderly, a study [17] revealed that 8% of females and 16% of males had developed ulcers before the age of 30 years.

AETIOLOGY

The major cause of leg ulceration is vascular insufficiency. A study of 357 patients with a total of 425 leg ulcers found 80% had some evidence of venous disease with nearly one third of patients having both an arterial and venous component [16]. Callam estimated between 60% and 80% of ulcerated legs will have evidence of venous disease [14].

Table 6.1 Types of leg ulcers

a.	Venous	Usually due to venous hypertension and characterized by variable sized ulcers over the medial and less frequently lateral malleoli may spread to involve whole gaiter area. Pigmentation of surrounding skin is common
b.	Arterial	These ulcers are usually due to tissue hypoxia and ischaemic changes due to occlusion of main vessels by atherosclerosis or thromboangitis obliterans. The ulcers are usually clearly defined with pale granulation tissue often covered by slough.
c.	Lymphatic	Small multiple ulcers prone to recurrent infections which destroy the lymphatic vessels associated with hyperplasia and thickening of the tissues
d.	Mixed	Often difficult to determine aetiology on inspection and examination due to presenting signs and symptoms

Ulcers less commonly seen

e1.	Immunological	Pyoderma gangrenosum, associated with ulcerative colitis. Presents as spontaneous gangrenous changes of the skin
e2.		Allergic vasculitis often appears as symmetrical red haemorrhagic papules with a central pustule and is associated with rheumatoid arthritis
e3.		Patients with a long-standing rheumatoid disease often develop ulcers that are difficult or non-healing
f.	Metabolic	Necrobiosis lipoidica diabeticorum, named because of its association with diabetes, can resemble a venous ulcer. Wound bed can appear as a glazed surface either red, yellow or brown in colour. Traversed by telangiectasis (dilated blood vessels)
f2.		Diabetic foot ulcers often as a result of neuropathic changes

Traumate/iatrogenic

g1.		These ulcers may be caused by physical, chemical or thermal damage, bites or stings, contact dermatitis, erythema pernio. Perhaps the most common cause, next to knocking the leg, is incorrect bandaging

Blood dyscrasias

h.		Blood dyscrasias associated with ulceration include haemolytic anaemia, sickle cell anaemia, polycythaemia vera, thrombotic thrombocythaemia, thalassaemia, myeloid metaplasia, cryoproteins

Table 6.1 *cont'd*

Infection

i.	Underlying causes include osteomyelitis, tropical ulcer, spirochaetal infection (yaws), syphilis, mycobacteriosis, leprosy, parasitosis, anthrax

Malignant

j1.	Squamous cell carcinoma (Marjolin's ulcer) may present as an irregular nodule, edges may be sloping
j2.	Basal cell carcinoma (rodent ulcer), more commonly found on the face than leg. The patient may give a history of repeated ulceration then healing, the tissue may appear bright red and bleed easily, the edges of the wound may be rolled
j3.	Kaposi's sarcoma (lymphangiosarcomas) present as small multiple reddish-purple lesions. Lesions are becoming more common and are associated with younger patients
j4.	Malignant melanoma are usually relatively easy to recognize

Approximately 10% of patients presenting with leg ulcers will have some degree of arterial insufficiency. Of the remaining ulcers, mixed aetiology will account for up to 15%, while lymphatic, immunological, metabolic, traumatic, iatrogenic, blood dyscrasias, infection and malignant factors form the more unusual and rarer causes. Table 6.1 summarizes the different types of ulcers.

PATHOPHYSIOLOGY OF VENOUS ULCERATION

The relationship between venous ulceration and the vascular system was first recorded by Hippocrates around 460–377 BC. He associated horse riding with varicosity of the veins because the feet, when riding, were always hanging down. He also noted that varicose veins did not occur before puberty [17].

The veins in the lower limbs consist of deep and superficial veins, separated by deep fascia and connected together by communicating veins, sometimes the term 'perforating' may be used. (Figures 6.1 and 6.2).

Blood is transported from the superficial veins to the deep veins via the communicator vein and then propelled towards the heart. The efficiency of the venous system is dependent upon the action

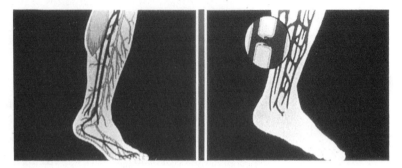

Figure 6.1 Venous stasis.

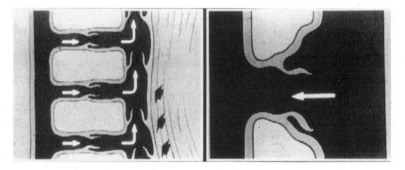

Figure 6.2 Venous stasis - detail.

of the ankle and calf muscle pump, the latter being referred to as the peripheral heart [2], due to its function.

Blood flows through the veins by the action of the surrounding muscle, which contracts and then relaxes. The direction of the flow is to a greater extent dependent upon the efficiency of the pumping mechanism and the competence of the valves inside the veins, which are designed to prevent backflow of the blood. The presence of the calf muscle pump was first noted in 1669 by Richard Lower.

Pressure in the venous system is normally low when a person is in the erect position whereas at rest the pressure at the ankle is between 70 and 100 mmHg, dropping to 0–30 mmHg on exercise and remaining at about 55 mmHg while sitting [18,19].

The valves of the leg veins are profuse and of great importance in the pump mechanism whereby in the upright position blood is returned to the heart against gravity [18].

Venous ulceration of the lower limb is primarily caused by venous hypertension and is associated with an elevated venous pressure in the legs when in the upright position and during exercise. Venous hypertension is the underlying cause of chronic venous insufficiency [8]. If the deep veins are obstructed or incompetence of the valves occurs as a result of deep vein thrombosis, degenerative or age related changes, congenital abnormalities or impairment of the calf muscle pump, then venous insufficiency can develop [9]. This causes a rise in the pressure within the veins during exercise and when in an erect position, due to a reflux action between the superficial veins and the communicator and soft or deep veins which appears to affect the intracapillary pressure in the skin [20], causing the endothelial pores to enlarge and capillary leakage to occur [21, 22] . This causes a change in the physiological status of the veins and capillaries which results in localized oedema due to the osmotic pull of lipids and proteins present in the interstitial fluid. The characteristic brown staining or pigmentation of the dermal cells is due to the breakdown of extra-vasated red blood cells.

Extravasation into the interstitial tissues of larger protein and lipid molecules causes fibrotic changes to occur in the affected limb and is commonly referred to as lipodermatosclerosis. Constriction of the tissues around the ankle gives the familiar 'champagne bottle' appearance to the leg.

The effect of venous hypertension on the microcirculation of the skin has been the topic of much debate. Three theories that have been postulated include:

1. fibrin cuff theory – Browse and Burnard (1982) [21]
2. white cell entrapment theory – Coleridge Smith *et al*. (1983) [23]
3. microthrombosis theory – Ehrly and Partsch (1989) [24]

FIBRIN CUFF THEORY

Browse and Burnard suggest there is physiological and patho-logical evidence [25, 26] to support the theory of fibrinogen leaking from the dilated capillaries and forming a pericapillary fibrin cuff which then prevents the diffusion of blood oxygen to the tissues. This hypothesis does not explain the whole story [17] as the lipo-dermatosclerosis is by no means invariably followed by ulceration and venous ulcers are not always surrounded by noticeable liposclerotic skin.

WHITE CELL ENTRAPMENT THEORY

This theory is based on the premise that white cells become trapped and accumulate in the circulation of dependent legs of patients with venous insufficiency [23, 27]; a visible reduction in the number of functioning capillary loops has also been noted in these patients [27].

It is suggested that the trapped white cells release proteolytic enzymes and toxic metabolites resulting in localized tissue necrosis and ulceration due to ischaemia [23, 27].

MICROTHROMBOSIS

The third theory, of microthrombi formation in the underlying vascular bed thereby impeding tissue perfusion, is less well known.

The precise mechanism by which venous hypertension causes ulceration remains unclear. Recent research suggests that many pathological processes are involved [28, 29] and it has even been suggested that the white cell theory and the fibrin cuff theory form different parts of the same phenomenon [30].

Venous ulceration may occur spontaneously or following trauma. It most commonly occurs on the medial aspect of the malleoli and may extend above the gaiter (midcalf) area. The wound edges are usually shallow and exudation can be quite profuse.

Many patients with venous ulcers complain of varying degrees of pain, often exacerbated by resting with the legs dependent.

Factors which may predispose a person to venous hypertension and ulceration include:

- Age – ulceration is more commonly found in the elderly population [4, 2].
- Sex – women are twice as likely to be affected as men [4, 2].
- Heredity – some evidence suggests familial tendencies towards anatomical abnormalities of the veins or valves [4, 18, 31–3].
- Race – there appears to be no conclusive evidence that race predisposes to ulceration. The lower incidence rate in African tribes is thought more likely to be a reflection of the different lifestyles between Western and African races [2, 18, 34]
- Hormonal – there is some evidence to suggest that a link between the development of varicose veins and hormonal levels exists [4, 18].
- Pregnancy and parity – in addition to hormonal changes, pressure on the iliac veins from the developing foetus is considered a causation factor.
- Diet – a lack of fibre combined with straining at defecation is thought to raise venous pressures [4, 35].

- Occupation – occupations involving sitting or standing for long periods of time increase the risk of venous hypertension [4].
- Environment, clothing and weight – the effects of extremes of temperature and the wearing of tight clothing such as corsets or gaiters are inconclusive, as are issues of weight. However, the wearing of tight footwear is widely acknowledged to cause pressure ulcers especially in patients with neuropathy.

Table 6.2 Venous ulceration

Clinical signs and symptoms	
Varicose veins	Varicosities vary in size and shape, defined as dilated tortuous veins with incompetent valves NB: Absence of varicose veins does not preclude a venous ulceration
Mild oedema	Around the ankle
Ankle flare	Dilated intradermal and subdermal venules around ankle, usually below medial malleolus
Pigmentation	Staining of the skin around ulcer site due to extravasation of red blood cells
Lipodermatosclerosis	Thickening and hardening of the dermis and subcutaneous tissue; 'champagne leg' develops due to fibrotic changes
Venous eczema/dermatitis	Eruption of the skin surrounding the ulcers by rash, usually weeping
Atrophe blanche	Appears as shiny white or ivory tissue stippled with red dots (capillary loops can appear without ulceration having been present)
Site of ulcer	Most commonly found near medial malleolus but can appear anywhere on lower limb
Subjective symptoms	
Itching	Especially over vein though may be no actual visible signs
Achiness or heaviness of legs	May be localized or more widely disseminated through leg
Pain	Often quite severe especially if legs dependent
Ulcer appearance	
Size and shape	Shallow, either round, oval or irregular in shape
Tissue at wound base	May be red granulation tissue or pale and unhealthy due to fibrotic changes associated with long standing
Ulceration	Slough may be present

CLINICAL FINDINGS

Assessment of the presenting clinical signs and symptoms of the ulcers (Table 6.2), when combined with findings from a comprehensive patient history and simple vascular assessment (Tables 6.3 and 6.4), will normally yield sufficient information to enable the nurse to make a diagnosis. If there is any doubt about the assessment findings or the nurse is at all concerned about the patient's progress or lack of it, the patient should be referred for a more detailed examination either by the general practitioner or appropriate clinical specialist (Table 6.5).

The use of Doppler ultrasound to assess the patient's resting pressure index as part of the vascular assessment has become more frequent both in hospital and community. The blood flow velocity is detected and registered as an audible sound. The resting pressure index is calculated by dividing the ankle pressure by the brachial pressure:

$$RPI = \frac{\text{Ankle systolic pressure}}{\text{Brachial systolic pressure}}$$

The resting pressure index should normally be greater than 1.0 mmHg.

In patients with venous hypertension compression therapy can be used if the pressure index is greater than 0.8 mmHg. If the reading is less than 0.8 mmHg compression therapy must not be used as arterial occlusion can arise. A pressure difference of between 0.5 and 0.75 mmHg indicates marked ischaemia and is usually associated with intermittent claudication.

Table 6.3 Simple vascular assessment

- Palpation of foot pulses:

  dorsalis pedis
  posterior tibial
  popliteal
  femoral

- Temperature assessment of feet and limbs (a heat gradient may be evident; patients with arterial problems are prone to cold limbs)
- Elevation of limbs above level of heart (colour of limb may change to pale if arterial insufficiency present)
- Blanching of toenail bed by direct pressure (colour should return within three seconds; if not, suspect arterial insufficiency)
- Muscle bulk (wasting of the calf muscle may be associated with arterial disease)
- Skin and hair (loss of hair, atrophic and shiny white skin are frequently present on patients with arterial disease)
- Stemmer's assessment (the ability to pick up skin over the metatarsophalangeal joint shows the absence of significant lymphoedema)
- Doppler assessment

Table 6.4 Assessment of the Patients Resting Pressure Index (based on work by C. Moffat, Leg Ulcer Specialist, Charing Cross Hospital, London)

1. The patient should lie down or sit with the legs elevated for 20 minutes.
2. Apply a sphygmomanometer cuff around patient's arm (as when taking the blood pressure).
3. Apply ultrasound gel over brachial pulse. Always use sufficient gel otherwise air will interfere with the transmission of sound.
4. Place Doppler probe gently over brachial pulse at an angle of 45° until a clear signal is heard.
5. Inflate cuff until the Doppler signal disappears. Then slowly reduce pressure until the signal returns. The return of signal is the brachial systolic pressure.
6. Palpate the foot for the posterior tibial and dorsalis pedis pulse or use the Doppler probe following the application of ultrasound gel.
7. Secure the sphygmomanometer cuff just above the malleolar area (above the ulcer). Inflate the cuff as above until the signal disappears. Then gradually reduce the pressure until the signal returns. The return of the signal signifies the ankle systolic pressure.
8. To calculate the pressure index, divide the ankle pressure by the brachial pressure.

Table 6.5 Additional vascular assessment techniques

Non-invasive

- Venous occlusion tests
- Thermography
- Photoplethysmography
- Foot volumetry

Invasive

- Foot vein pressure measurements
- Femoral vein pressure measurements
- Femoral artery pressure measurements
- Arteriography
- Venography

TREATMENT OPTIONS

The actual management of the ulcers should be determined by the characteristics of the patient's wound, surrounding skin and priorities for care. The most important aspect of leg ulcer management relates to treating the underlying cause. For some patients surgical intervention may prevent further recurrence of the ulcer. However, efforts to restore valvular function to deep veins have shown poor results or at best indifferent long term results [18]. It is suggested that surgery for the treatment of leg ulcers be limited to communicator vein ligation and saphenous ligation and stripping with patients being advised to wear kneelength firm compression stockings when ambulant [18].

Plastic surgery has been successful for some patients. The choice between a split skin or pinch graft is a clinical decision but many surgeons appear to favour the use of pinch grafts.

CONSERVATIVE MANAGEMENT

The main aim of conservative management for patients with venous ulceration is to reverse the effects of venous and capillary hypertension. There is a substantial body of research to support claims that sustained graduated compression provides an optimum therapeutic environment [12, 36–40]. By increasing the transfer of tissue fluid from the interstitial spaces back into the vascular and lymphatic compartments and achieving a maximal increase in venous velocity in order to reduce pooling of blood in the calf veins, healing of the venous ulcers may be enhanced [40].

Compression therapy is also suitable for most patients with oedema, lymphoedema and varicose veins.

Compression bandages are designed to extend and maintain sustained pressure beneath the bandage. The degree of pressure required should be determined by the condition to be treated. When considering which bandage regime to use it is important to remember that pressure is directly proportional to the number of layers and the tension created on application of the bandage and inversely proportional to the diameter of the limb and width of the bandage. This equation is termed Laplace's Law and may be expressed as:

$$P = \frac{T \times N \times 4630}{C \times W}$$

where

P = pressure (in mmHg)
T = bandage tension (in kg)
C = circumference of the limb (in cm)
W = bandage width (in cm)
N = number of layers applied.

An external ankle pressure of 35–40 mmHg is generally accepted as the minimal pressure required to prevent capillary leakage and reverse venous hypertension. In patients with severe lymphoedema or with an ankle circumference greater than 23 cm, higher pressures may be required.

Compression bandages are classified into four compression groups: light, moderate, high and extra high (Table 6.6). Difficulties have been reported in sustaining compression with some bandages, with one quarter of the initial pressure dissipating within 30 minutes under

Table 6.6 Compression bandages

Short stretch (maintain their position when the calf muscle expands)	Rosidal K (Lohmann) Comprilan (BDF)
Long stretch (stretch as the calf muscle expands)	Bilastic (Forte) Blue Line (Seton) Elastoweb (Smith & Nephew) Setopress (Seton) Tensopress (Smith & Nephew) Veinopress - Steriseal Elastocrepe (Smith & Nephew) Litepress (Smith & Nephew)

adhesive plaster bandages and three quarters of the pressure dissipating under a single elastic bandage within eight hours [13, 41–3].

Interest in understanding and applying the principles of compression bandaging has witnessed a recent revival and heralded the introduction of several new bandages and bandage systems; Table 6.7 gives examples. Light support and cohesion bandages have been used in conjunction with other bandages in the four layer bandage system developed at Charing Cross [53] to sustain graduated compression (Table 6.8).

Light support bandages are designed to provide support and prevent the formation of oedema following traumatic injury such as sprains and strains. Support bandages are often made of British Pharmacopoeia (BP) 'crepe' based woven cotton products. These bandages are generally considered unsuitable in the treatment of venous hypertension despite their continuing use, as they do not usually apply or maintain clinically acceptable levels of compression.

Adhesive bandages have an adhesive coating applied to either woven cotton or viscose and cotton. These bandages adhere to the skin and tend to remain *in situ*, so they are not usually applied to very friable skin as trauma may arise on removal.

Cohesive bandages adhere to themselves due to a special coating, so they are especially useful in helping to prevent slippage of other bandages.

Table 6.7 Light support and cohesive bandages

Light support	Crepe
Cohesive	Coban (3M) Secure Forte (Johnson & Johnson) Lestroflex (Seton) Co-plus (Smith & Nephew)

Table 6.8 4 layer bandage system for venous
ulcers based on ankle circumference [53]

18 cm or less	18–25 cm
2 or more Velband	1 Velband
1 Crepe	1 Crepe
1 Elset	1 Elset
1 Coban	1 Coban
25–30 cm	**more than 30 cm**
1 Velban	1 Velband
1 Plastex 23	1 Elset
1 Coban	1 Plastex 23
	1 Coban

PASTE BANDAGES

There are five groups of medicated paste bandages currently available
in the United Kingdom; most contain zinc oxide. All paste bandages
require a secondary dressing and are designed to treat specific skin
conditions associated with ulceration of the lower limbs, not the actual
ulcer. For ease of reference the information has been produced in Table
6.9.

Paste bandages tend to be used more frequently in the community
than in hospital. As with all products, practitioners should familiarize
themselves with the manufacturer's instructions on selection, application and removal of these bandages. Many of the bandages can be
left up to two weeks *in situ*. It should be remembered that all paste
bandages contain preservatives so the longer they are used by the
patient, the greater the risk of sensitivity due to the accumulation of
the parabens under the skin.

A paste bandage in conjunction with a short stretch bandage has
been used successfully to treat some patients who present with a
dermatological problem and venous hypertension.

ELASTIC COMPRESSION HOSIERY

Many patients are unable to wear or do not require a compression bandage as part of their treatment programme. Hence a range
of elastic compression stockings are available. The greatest compression is obtained at the ankle, as with compression bandages
(Table 6.10).

Three different classes of stocking have been included on the drug
tariff in the United Kingdom. The stockings described as graduated

Table 6.9 Criteria for use of a paste bandage

Skin condition	Type of paste bandage	Anticipated actions
Inflamed and sensitive	• Zinc paste • Viscopaste PB7 (Smith & Nephew) • Zincoband (Seton) (both bandages contain parabens)	Soothes and protects sensitive skin
Lichenification (dry scaly skin), eczema, atopic dermatitis	• Zinc paste and coal tar • Tarband (Seton) (contains lanolin) • Caltopaste (Smith & Nephew) (contains parabens)	Improves condition of skin. For short term use only as a bandage may interrupt granulation process
Moist eczema	• Zinc paste and ichthammol • Ichthopaste (Smith & Nephew) (contains gelatin) • Ichthoband (Seton) (contains parabens)	Soothes and has an anti-inflammatory action. Useful for patients who cannot tolerate coal tar
Clinically infected malodorous leg ulcers	• Zinc paste, calamine and cliquinol • Quinaband (Seton)	Mild antibacterial activity reduces odour and combats infection
Fragile skin with acute/subacute eczema	• Zinc paste and calamine	Soothes inflamed, irritated fragile skin
Dermatitis	Calaband (Seton)	

Table 6.10 Compression elastic hosiery

Ankle compression	Class	Type	Indication
14-17 mmHg	1	Light	Superficial varicose veins, mild oedema, venous ulcers
18-24 mmHg	2	Medium	Prevention and treatment post vein surgery. Moderate varices
25-35 mmHg	3	Strong	Severe varicose veins, ankle oedema. Lymphatic disorders, venous ulceration

Table 6.11 British Standard Specification (BS 6612:1985)

Type	BSS	(Switzerland) SIGVARIS	Germany
Light	14-17	20-30	18-21
Medium	18-24	30-40	25-32
Strong	25-35	40-50	36-46
Very strong		50-60	59

Represent:
The Association of Manufacturers of Medical Elastic Stockings and the German Society for Phlebology and Proctology categorization of hosiery (rounded into the nearest whole number)

compression hosiery comply to the British Standard Specification (BS 6612:1985) (Table 6.11). The same criteria are applied to compression bandages.

Stockings are also available in this country that are made to Swiss and German specification, although many are not available on the drug tariff (Table 6.11). Some manufacturers produce coloured kneelength stockings which are often preferred by men. For patients who have difficulty in applying their hosiery, Medi (UK) have produced a very useful stocking valet. Another recent innovation has been the introduction of a zip sewn in the back of the stocking.

SHAPED ELASTICATED TUBULAR BANDAGES

Shaped elasticated tubular bandages also provide graduated compression, albeit at a very low pressure. They are extremely useful for patients who are unable to tolerate a compression bandage or who require a greater level of dependence than achievable by wearing a compression bandage.

Practical considerations when selecting a compression bandage or hosiery should include:

- suitability for the purpose intended;
- ease of application and removal, especially over a dressing;
- maintenance of compression therapy;
- patient comfort and compliance;
- ability to wash without loss of function (unless once-only use);
- conformability;
- wearable without modification to footwear or clothing;
- availability;
- efficacy and safety;
- cost effectiveness.

It is important to reassess and measure the patient's limb size, especially if oedema or lymphoedema is present, as a reduction in limb size will affect the efficacy of the product. Patients should always be given written guidelines and instructions on how to care for their lower limbs and bandages/hosiery correctly, in addition to general health advice on how to promote wound healing and prevent recurrence of the ulcer.

SEQUENTIAL COMPRESSION THERAPY (SCT)

Sequential compression therapy is also known as intermittent sequential pneumatic compression and is derived from the principles of pneumotherapy (compressing limbs in air bags) to reduce oedema [45]. Reference has been made to the application of this technique in the prevention of deep vein thrombosis [46, 47].

More recently, interest has developed in the application of SCT in the treatment of leg ulcers [48–52]. Treatment is by using multichambered garments that fill in turn with compressed air. The first and second chambers fill and as the third chamber commences to fill, air is transferred from the first chamber to the third and so on up the length of the garment, creating a peristaltic action. The cycle is repeated for the duration of the treatment period with each cell being inflated for a period of 4–12 seconds. Depending upon the cycle time set on the machine, varying pressures can be supplied. A light massage can be achieved by using a 40 second cycle, a 60 second cycle deepens the massage whereas a 120 second cycle gives a deep penetrating massage. The effect of this massage appears to push fluid from the interstitial spaces into the venous and lymphatic vessels, thus reducing oedema. The peristaltic motion acts as an effleurage and is thought to stimulate the vascular system, thereby improving oxygenation and perfusion of the tissues and facilitating the removal of waste products.

A range of garments and machines is currently available to treat a wide variety of conditions including lymphoedema, oedema and sports injuries. It is used pre- and postsurgery to improve the circulation and reduce the risk of deep vein thrombosis, oedema following a cerebrovascular accident or to enhance mobility in patients with conditions such as multiple sclerosis and peripheral neuritis.

Further investigation is in progress to identify the precise action of SCT in patients with venous ulceration.

PHARMACOKINETIC THERAPY

The use of pharmacological agents in the treatment of venous ulceration is still in its infancy. Much work needs to be undertaken before there is sufficient research evidence upon which the practitioner can base their decision. Table 6.12 gives an overview of some of the agents that are being investigated in the management of vascular insufficiency of the lower limbs.

However, all pharmacological agents must be used in conjunction with compression hosiery or bandages for the treatment of venous hypertension.

Table 6.12 Pharmacokinetic agents

Drug	Possible indication	Action
Stanozolol (Stromba)	• Lipodermatosclerosis (acute) • Venous ulceration	Enhances fibrinolytic action Mild anabolic steroid
Oxpentyfylline (Trental)	• Ischaemic ulceration (good results) • Venous ulceration • Peripheral vascular disease	Aggregation of leucocytes inhibited Enhances fibrinolytic action
(Venoruton) Paroven Hyroxyrutosides	• Oedematous limb • Venous insufficiency • Venous ulceration	Improves the microcirculation by reducing capillary permeability
Defibrontide	• Lipodermatosclerosis • Venous hypertension • Venous ulceration	Antithrombosis agent and enhances fibrinolytic action
Prostaglandins	• Ischaemic ulceration • Venous ulceration	Aggregation of platelets inhibited. Reduction of rest pain. Vasodilation

The use of sclerosing agents injected into the superficial veins as a treatment for varicosities has produced poor results in many patients and has not prevented further ulceration nor the recurrence of varices.

Diuretics may be prescribed for patients to enhance the removal of excess fluid, thereby reducing limb oedema as part of the patient's general management. The use of growth factors is still at an early stage of development (Chapter 1).

PAIN MANAGEMENT

According to many patients with leg ulcers, effective pain control is difficult if not at times impossible to achieve. The pain experienced is not limited to one specific type of ulcer.

Pain indicates a potential threat to a person's control over the situation in which the pain has occurred and possible future events. The degree of perceived threat and hence anxiety depends upon the pain sensation, the information available about the nature, cause and potential consequences of the pain and the individual's interpretation of this information in relation to their existing knowledge and past experience.

Many patients with chronic pain undergo a process of physical and psychological adaptation. Walker [44] identified a range of negative and positive responses to the presence of chronic pain (Chapter 3 and 7). There are only a limited number of potential outcomes to a painful event which are determined by healing processes and available coping resources. The latter comprise personal, social and medical factors including personality and attitude, available social and practical support and availability of effective medical or alternative pain treatments. The application of moist wound healing principles has been found to reduce pain at the wound site for many patients. An atraumatic removal and application of a dressing also reduces the incidence of local pain. It is beyond the scope of this book to provide a detailed account of pain and methods of control.

ARTERIAL ULCERS

Arterial ulcers are a direct result of tissue hypoxia and necrosis due to arterial insufficiency. The main cause of this condition is atherosclerosis of the arteries, often associated with underlying pathological conditions such as diabetes, Buerger's or Raynaud's disease. Factors which may predispose to atherosclerosis include smoking (Table 6.13). Arterial occlusion due to emboli can occur, but usually tends to be associated with a rapid and extremely painful deterioration of the affected leg.

Table 6.13 Factors predisposing to atherosclerosis

Smoking	Thomas found 90% of patients with chronic ischaemic limbs were smokers
Hyperlipidaemia	A link between atherosclerosis and hyperlipidaemia has been indicated due to damage to the vascular endothelium
Cholesterol	Blist highlighted that 38% of atherosclerotic patients with raised cholesterol had arterial disease of the lower limbs. Other researchers found a reduction in HDL and cholesterol levels
Diabetes	Abnormal glucose tolerance tests have been found by Blist in patients with ischaemic disease of the lower limbs
Stress	Biochemical changes as a result of social or economic stress predisposed to atherosclerosis
Hormones	Research indicates a clear link between oestrogen levels and the development of atherosclerosis

Many people may have the signs of arterial insufficiency for many years without an ulcer developing. Repeated trauma from ill fitting footwear, poor foot hygiene, misuse of hot water bottles, sitting too close to the fire and banging into objects often precipitate ulceration. Clinical signs and symptoms associated with arterial ulceration are given in Table 6.14.

Unfortunately, once developed, arterial ulcers can be extremely difficult to heal due to poor tissue perfusion. The wound's requirement for oxygen to aid healing creates an even greater hypoxic effect resulting in an extension of the lesion. The majority of arterial ulcers are usually found on the lateral aspect of the leg or foot, but not always.

Patients with arterial insufficiency often complain of severe cramplike pain in the calf muscle region which may be precipitated by activity. Some patients experience a constant ache even when resting, especially if the legs are elevated. Pain may be localized in the foot or toes. This situation frequently occurs at night, requiring the patient to spend the night sitting with the legs dependent in a chair.

Practitioners should remember that patients with a neuropathy may have diminished pain sensation which may increase the risk of further trauma. A detailed pain assessment and treatment regime should be devised to alleviate/minimize pain.

Table 6.14 Signs and symptoms of arterial ulceration

Signs

- Cooling or coldness of foot or limb (temperature gradient may be evident)
- Atrophic shiny skin
- Muscle wasting
- Absence of hair
- Onychogryphosis (overgrowth of the nails)
- Slow return of colour (> 3 s) after nail blanching test
- Pallor, cyanosis and blotchy erythema are evidence of arterial insufficiency
- Marked pallor when limb elevated
- Weak or absent pedal and/or dorsalis pedis pulses
- Paresis of devitalized tissue (heralding necrosis)

Symptoms

Pain on exercise - severe arterial insufficiency - results in intermittent claudication

Ulcer characteristics

Size and shape	Deep irregular shaped lesion, edges often appear punched out. Frequently on the lateral aspect of the leg or foot
Tissue at wound bed	May be pale and unhealthy due to fibrotic changes associated with long-standing ulceration. Slough is frequently present.

TREATMENT OPTIONS

Following assessment and documentation the needs of the wound should be addressed and a suitable management regime introduced to promote an ideal environment for healing. Compression must not be applied to an ischaemic ulcer, with an ankle pressure index of less than 0.8 mmHg.

Revascularization may be an option for some patients whereas others may benefit from plastic surgery, combined with good medical management.

General care guidelines should include:

- special attention to the skin between the toes;
- regular visits to the chiropodist
- avoiding infections of the skin and nail bed;
- good personal hygiene especially to the feet;
- wearing of well fitting footwear;
- not wearing garters;
- keeping the skin hydrated;

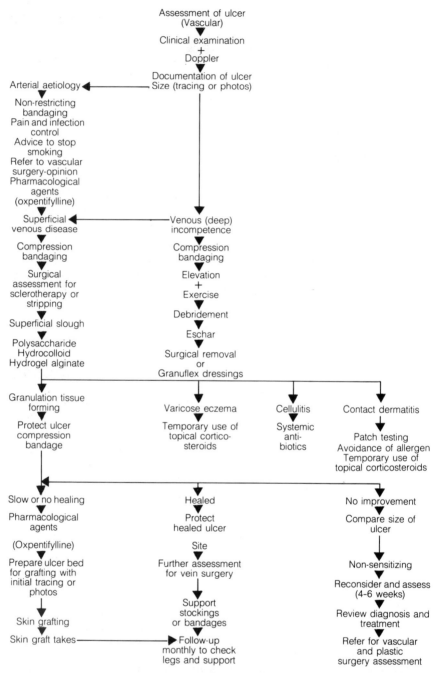

The importance of proper vascular assessment is essential in successful leg ulcer management. The flow charge that we have developed for treating leg ulcers begins with vascular assessment of the legs

Figure 6.3 Oxford flowchart for the management of leg ulcers. Reproduced by kind permission from Dr G. Cherry, modified by M. Moody and G. Bennett.

- not using hot water bottles or electric blankets;
- maintaining a good posture, not crossing legs;
- reducing the intake of saturated fats/alcohol;
- increasing the intake of vitamins;
- not smoking.

MIXED AETIOLOGY ULCERS

As indicated in Table 6.1, some patients present with ulcers that are of mixed aetiology. A high proportion of elderly patients appear to have a combination of venous hypertension and arterial insufficiency. Others may present with involvement of the lymphatic system or as a result of an underlying immunological, metabolic or haematological condition. An infection or traumatic experience can also result in ulceration.

Malignant ulcers, although considered rare, need early recognition and treatment if extensive tissue damage and poor prognosis are to be avoided. Some lesions are likely to become more common and be associated with younger patients who develop lymphangiosarcomas.

Management should always be based on analysis of the assessment findings, patient priorities and attainment of achievable outcomes. The development of flow charts is one simple way to highlight treatment options (Figure 6.3).

Accurate documentation of information combined with evaluation of the management outcomes are essential prerequisites of quality based patient care.

As practitioners we should be aware of the patient's perception of the leg ulcer and the impact leg ulcers have on lifestyle [54].

REFERENCES

1. Major, R.H. (1854) *A History of Medicine, vol. 1*, Blackwell, Oxford.
2. Browse, N.I., Burnard, K.G. and Thomas, M.L. (1988) *Diseases of the Veins: Pathology, Diagnosis and Treatment*, Edward Arnold, London.
3. Laing, W. (1992). *Chronic Venous Diseases of the Leg*, Office of Health Economics, London.
4. Department of Health (1989) *Projected Changes in Population England 1989–2000*, Office of Population Censuses and Surveys, London.
5. Wilson, E. (1989). Prevention and treatment of venous leg ulcers. *Health Trends*, **21**, 97.
6. Bosanquet, N. (1992) Costs of venous ulcers; from maintenance to therapy to investment programmes. *Phlebology*, **7** (suppl.), 44–6.
7. Dale, J. and Gibson, B. (1986) The epidemiology of leg ulcers. *Prof. Nurse*, **1**(8), 215–16.
8. Cornwell, J., Dore, C. and Lewis, J. (1986) Leg ulcers: epidemiology and aetiology. *Br J Surg*, **73**, 693–6.

9. Hunt, S. (1982) Subjective health of patients with peripheral vascular disease. *Practitioner*, **226**, 133–6.
10. Callum, M., Dale, J., Harper, D. and Ruckley, C. (1987) Arterial diseases in chronic leg ulcerations: an underestimated hazard. Lowthian and Forth Valley leg ulcer study. *Br Med J*, **294**, 929–31.
11. Moody, M. (1993). Salisbury Health Care Leg Ulcer Survey. Unpublished survey for Salisbury Health Care, Salisbury, Wiltshire.
12. Morison, M.J. and Moffat, C. (1994) *A Colour Guide to the Assessment and Management of Leg Ulcers*, 2nd edn, Mosby International, London.
13. Elizalde, J.M.A. (1992) Vascular ulcers of the lower limb, in *Advanced Wound Healing Resource Pack*, (ed. K.Harting), Coloplast (UK), Peterborough.
14. Callam, M. (1992) Prevalence of chronic leg ulceration and severe chronic venous disease in Western Countries. *Phlebology*, **7** (suppl.), 6–12.
15. Callam, M.J., Ruckley, C.V., Harper, D.R. and Dale, J.R. (1985) Chronic ulceration of the leg: extent of the problem and provision. *Br Med J*, **290**, 1855–6.
16. Cornwell, J. and Lewis, J. (1983) Leg ulcer revisited. *Br J Surg*, **70**, 681.
17. Negus, D. (1991) *Leg Ulcers: A Practical Approach to Management*, Butterworth Heinemann, Oxford.
18. Dodd, H. and Cockett, F.B. (1976) *The Pathology and Surgery of Veins of the Lower Limb*, Churchill Livingstone, London.
19. Ryan, T.J. and Wilkinson, D. (1984) Diseases of the veins and arteries – leg ulcers, in *Textbook of Dermatology*, (eds R. Champion, J. Burton and F. Ebling), Blackwell Scientific, Oxford, pp. 1187–208.
20. Burnard, K.G., Whimster, I., Clemenson, G. *et al.* (1981) The relationship between the number of capillaries in the skin of the venous ulcer – bearing area of the lower leg and the fall in foot vein pressure during exercise. *Br J Surg*, **68**, 297–300.
21. Browse, N.L., Burnard, K.G. (1982) The cause of venous ulceration: hypothesis, *Lancet*, **11**, 243–5.
22. Brunard, K.G., Whimster, I., Maidoo, A. and Browse, N.L. (1982) Pericapillary fibrin in the ulcer-bearing skin of the leg: the cause of lipodermatosclerosis and venous ulceration. *Br Med J*, **285**, 1071–2.
23. Coleridge Smith, P.D., Thomas, P., Scurr, J.H. and Dormandy, J.A. (1988) Causes of venous ulceration: a new hypothesis. *Br Med J*, **296**, 1726–7.
24. Ehrly, A.M. and Partsch, H. (1989) Microcirculatory and haemorrhalogical abnormalities in venous leg ulcers: introductory remarks, in *Phlebologie* (eds A. Davy and R. Stemmer), Libbey, Paris, pp. 142–5.
25. Blalock, A. (1929) Oxygen content of blood in patients with varicose veins. *Arch Surg*, **19**, 898–905.
26. Hopkins, N.F.G., Spinks, T.J., Rhodes, C.G., Ranicar, A.S.O. and Jamieson, C.W.(1913) Positron emission tomography in venous ulceration and liposclerosis: study of regional tissue function. *Br Med J*, 286–333.
27. Thomas, P.R.S., Nash, G.B. and Dormandy, J.A. (1988) White cell accumulation in dependent legs of patients with venous hypertension: a possible mechanism for trophic changes in the skin. *Br Med J*, **296**, 1693–5.

28. Scott, H.J., McMullin, G.H., Coleridge Smith, P.D. and Scurr, J.S. (1989) The microcirculation and venous ulceration in the skin of the calf, in *Phlebologie*, (eds A. Davy and R. Stemmer), Libbey, Paris, pp. 282–4.

29. Scurr, J.H. and Coleridge Smith, P.D. (1992) Pathogenesis of venous ulceration. *Phlebology*, (suppl.), **7**, 13–15.

30. Herrick, S.E., Sloan, P, McGurk, M., Freak, L., McCollum, C.N. and Ferguson, M.W.J. (1992) Sequential changes in histological pattern and cellular matrix deposition during the healing of chronic venous ulcers 17n. *J Pathol*, **141**(5), 1085–95.

31. Basmajian, J.V. (1952) The distribution of valves in the femoral, external iliac, and common femoral veins and their relationship of varicose veins. *Surg Gynecol Obstet*, **95**, 537–9.

32. Powell, T. and Lynn, R.B. (1951) The valves of the external iliac, femoral, and upper third of the popliteal veins. *Surg Gynecol Obstet*, **92**, 453–7.

33. Reagan, B. and Folse, R. (1971) Lower limb venous dynamics in normal persons and children or patients with varicose veins. *Surg Gynecol Obstet*, **132**, 15–18.

34. Dodd, H.J. (1964) The cause, prevention and arrest of varicose veins. *Lancet*, **2**, 809.

35. Burkitt, D.P. (1972) Varicose veins, deep vein thrombosis and haemorrhoids: epidemiology and suggested aetiology. *Br Med J*, **2**, 556.

36. Frank, A. (1993) Vascular assessment of wounds: theory and practice. *Wound Man*, **43**, 72–5.

37. Stemmer, R. Compression treatments of the lower extremities with compression stocking. *Dermatologists*, **31**, 355–65.

38. Blair, S.D., Wright, D.D.I., Blackhouse, C.M, Riddle, E.M. and McCallum, C.W. (1988) Sustained compression and healing of chronic venous ulcer. *Br Med J*, **297**, 1159–61.

39. Sockalingham, S., Barbenel, J.C. and Queen, D. (1990) Ambulatory monitoring of the pressures beneath compression bandages. *Care Sc Pract*, **8**, 56–60.

40. Thomas, S. (1990) Bandages and bandaging, in *Wound Management and Dressings*, (ed. Thomas, S.), Pharmaceutical Press, London.

41. Thomas, S. (1990) Bandages and bandaging: the science behind the art. *Care Sci Pract*, **8**(2), 56–60.

42. Ray, T.B., Goddard, M. and Makin, G.C. (1980) How long do compression bandages maintain their pressure during ambulatory treatment of varicose veins? *Br J Surg*, **67**, 122–4.

43. Dale, J.J., Callum, M.J. and Ruckley, C.V. (1983) How sufficient is a compression bandage? *Nursing Times*, **79**(46), 49–51.

44. Walker, J.M. (1989) The management of elderly patients with pain: a community nursing prospective. Doctoral thesis, Nursing and Health Care Research Unit, Dorset Institute (now Institute of Health and Community Services), University of Bournemouth.

45. Pflugh, J.J. (1975) Intermittent compression of the swollen leg in general practice. *Practitioner*, **215**, 69.

46. Hills, N.H., Pflugh, J.J., Jeyasingh, K, Beardman, L. and Calman, J.S. (1972) Prevention of deep vein thrombosis by intermittent compression of the calf. *Br Med J*, **1**, 131.

47. Nicholaides, A.N., Fernandes, J. and Fernandes, J., Pollock, A.V. (1980) Intermittent sequential pneumatic compression of the legs in the prevention of venous stasis and postoperative deep venous thrombosis surgery. *Surgery*, **87**(1), 69–76.

48. Zelikowski, A., Argranant, A., Sternberg, A., Haddad, M. and Urca, I. (1978) The conservative treatment of stasis ulcers. *Angiology*, **29**, 832.

49. Hazarika, E.X. and Wright, D.E. (1981) Chronic leg ulcers: the effect of pneumatic intermittent compression. *Practitioner*, **255**, 189–92.

50. Belcaro, G.V. and Coen, F. (1986) Pneumatic intermittent compression treatment of venous ulceration caused by hypertension, in *Phlebology*, (eds M. Negus, and D. Janlet), Libbey, Paris, p. 85.

51. Coleridge Smith, P.D, Hasty, J. and Scurr, J.H. (1990) Sequential gradient pneumatic compression enhances venous ulcer healing. A randomised trial. *Surgery*, **108**, 871–5.

52. Moody, M. and Slade, D. (1993) Role of sequential therapy in the treatment of vascular ulcers. *J Wound Care* (in press).

53. Moffatt, C. (1993) The Charing Cross high compression four layer bandage system. Update. *Wound Care*, **2**(2), 9–4.

54. Hamer, C., Cullum, V.A. and Rose, B.H. (1994) Patients' perceptions of chronic leg ulcers. *J Wound Care*, **3**(2), 99–101.

Management of complex and difficult to heal wounds 7

The majority of wounds, regardless of origin, heal uneventfully by a series of highly complex cellular and biochemical processes. Only a small proportion of wounds develop problems, but they can pose a significant challenge for both patient and carer.

Wounds may be designated as complex or difficult to heal for a variety of reasons. Advances in medical and nursing knowledge combined with new techniques of surgery and diagnostic assessment have done much to eliminate or reduce the incidents of postoperative complications such as haemorrhage, haematoma formation, clinical infection, wound dehiscence, fistula or sinus formation, adhesions and incisional hernia. The management of underlying metabolic disorders such as diabetes, uraemia and anaemia combined with a greater understanding of pharmacokinetics and the influence of drugs, for example to suppress the inflammatory process, have greatly enhanced patient care.

The introduction of modern dressings to create a local environment for optimum wound healing has helped to reduce the number of problem wounds by effectively treating wound characteristics that have a negative effect on healing such as the presence of necrotic tissue, slough and excessive exudation. Wounds to the eye, face, hand, foot, perianal and vulvar regions of the body are often associated with varying degrees of difficulty. The actual size of the wound can add to its complexity. The more extensive the tissue loss, the greater the challenge for the wound management team.

This chapter will give an overview of some of the complex and difficult to heal wounds frequently encountered by nurses and doctors that are not covered elsewhere in the text.

WOUND DEHISCENCE, FISTULA AND SINUS FORMATION

WOUND DEHISCENCE

The term wound dehiscence refers to the partial or complete separation of a surgical wound and was a common postoperative complication before improvements in pre-, peri- and postoperative procedures greatly reduced the incidence of wound infection and dehiscence.

The most frequent cause of this complication is inability of the suture material to hold the wound together until healing has progressed to a stage of self-sufficiency. Local predisposing factors include poor tissue perfusion, trauma to the surrounding tissues, incorrect apposition of wound edges, poor suturing technique, inadequate strength of suture material, foreign body and infection. Factors such as poor nutrition, age, obesity, dehydration, anaemia and other underlying conditions previously discussed can also increase the risk of wound dehiscence.

Separation of a wound with or without exposure of the viscera can be a frightening experience for both patient and nurse. If the viscera is exposed it should not be touched; the nurse must reassure the patient and cover the wound with a sterile damp towel and call the duty surgeon immediately. It may be helpful to ask the patient to bend their knees to relieve pressure. A record of the pulse and blood pressure should be kept and an intravenous infusion and antibiotics may be required. When the viscera is exposed emergency surgery is usually indicated.

FISTULA

A fistula is the term used to describe an abnormal tract of granulation tissue which connects one viscus to another or a viscus to the skin surface. Some patients may have a fistula deliberately created – gastrostomy, colostomy, nephrostomy – as part of a planned surgical intervention to alleviate or treat an underlying condition. Alternatively they may develop as a complication of a malignancy or chronic inflammatory condition of the bowel. Postoperative fistulae are usually due to a breakdown of an anastomosis or accidental damage of the viscus during the operative procedure. Only fistulae opening onto the skin surface will be discussed here.

The escape of secretions from the connecting viscus can, after analysis, provide the clinician with information to support a diagnosis (Table 7.1). Other investigations may include radiological assessment, the injection of dyes and analysis of the patient's blood urea, electrolytes, haemoglobin and serum proteins to facilitate early detection of biochemical imbalance and hypoproteinaemia.

Table 7.1 Secretions

Type of secretion	Origin of fistula	Comments
Watery	Gastric	Test with litmus paper - acidic may contain undigested food particles
Bile	Gastric Biliary Duodenum	Rapid excoriation of the skin
Yellow/orange	Small bowel	Rapid excoriation of surrounding skin due to enzyme action
Colourless	Pancreas	As above
Brown faecal	Large bowel	Often preceded by purulent discharge
Serosanginous	Abdomen Thoracic cavity	Usually associated with large volumes of fluid being produced

Priorities for the nurse must include protection of the patient's skin against excoriation. This requires efficient collection and containment of the secretions; the actual receptacle selected should be determined by the volume of fluid loss and the location of the fistula. Dehydration can rapidly develop if the patient is losing large volumes of fluid so fluid loss must be accurately measured and recorded. The use of products like Stomahesive applied to the skin surrounding the fistula has done much to improve local management and reduce and treat excoriation.

For most patients with a fistula the wound will heal spontaneously providing it is appropriately managed and they are not malnourished or dehydrated. Only a small proportion of these wounds fail to heal by conservative measures and these may include patients who have a malignant tumour or distal obstruction, persistent chronic inflammatory condition or epithelialization of the tract lining.

SINUS

A sinus is the term used to describe a non-healing blind-ended tract which communicates from the skin to an abscess cavity. All sinus cavities contain some form of foreign material which may include retained postoperative dressing or non-absorbable suture material, fragments of metal or glass, pieces of wood or plastic. Hair is known to be the causative factor in patients who develop a pilonidal sinus, so its presence in the tissues stimulates a marked inflammatory response and abscess formation. Patients with chronic osteomyelitis can develop sequestration of the bone which can give rise to a malodorous brown coloured discharge; this condition can occur as a complication of pressure sores. Chronic sinuses are often the reason for non-healing pressure sores, especially when associated with poor drainage and premature wound closure, thus providing an ideal environment for infection and abscess formation.

The primary aim of treatment is to drain the abscess and prevent recurrence and the exact procedure will be determined by the clinician. Some wounds may be closed after exploration and drainage with or without a drain *in situ*; others are left open. If the sinus cavity is excised and the wound left to heal by secondary intention, the local management is of paramount importance if the wound is to heal satisfactorily. The dressing selected should facilitate the removal of exudate, provide an optimum environment for healing and allow atraumatic application and removal so as to avoid all risk of damage to the newly forming tissue.

WOUNDS SEEN IN ACCIDENT AND EMERGENCY DEPARTMENTS

The management of wounds in the Accident and Emergency department is largely determined by their aetiology. Tissue damage sustained by contact with high or low velocity missiles is due to the transfer of energy from the missile to the tissues, the actual wounding capacity of the missile being directly proportional to its kinetic energy.

Low velocity missiles cause less tissue damage than high velocity missiles which have a tendency to create a large cavity approximately 30–40 times the diameter of the missile. The shock waves cause the tissues to accelerate violently forwards and outwards, creating a sub-atmospheric pressure due to an opening of the entry and exit point. The cavity rapidly collapses in a pulsatile fashion, sucking debris, bacteria and air into the wound, causing gross contamination.

Priorities of management include resuscitation, arrest of haemorrhage, debridement of dead, devitalized and contaminated tissue, systemic antibiotics to prevent a clinical infection and delayed primary closure of the wound some 4–5 days after the initial injury. The effects of bomb blast injuries can result in traumatic amputation of limbs due to the impact of pressure waves following the blast. Penetration injuries can result in injury to underlying organs and the introduction of foreign bodies. It is a useful rule never to remove knives or other transfixing missiles until the patient reaches the operating theatre. Wounds that sometimes appear to be trivial, such as minor cuts and abrasions, can lead to serious complications if foreign bodies are left undetected in the tissues. Careful inspection and cleansing of traumatic injuries is an essential prerequisite prior to suturing or application of the wound dressing. Avulsion or degloving injuries result in the sudden and traumatic separation of skin and fascia from the underlying blood supply, causing hypoxia and the subsequent development of ischaemia to the affected tissues. The primary aim of local management is restoration of the blood supply and the creation of an optimum environment to facilitate healing. Crush and contusion injuries can result in severe disruption of the microcirculation and lead to tissue hypoxia and necrosis.

Priorities for the management of acutely inflicted wounds are the same as for all wounds: arrest of haemorrhage, the promotion of good haemostasis, effective wound cleansing, debridement of dead or devitalized tissue, prevention of complications by detailed assessment, application of a dressing suitable for the wound's requirements and careful monitoring of the patient's progress.

DIABETIC FOOT ULCERATION

Prevention of ulceration is almost more important than treatment of the ulceration when it occurs [1]. Foot problems account for more days spent in hospital than any other complication of diabetes [2]. An understanding of the factors involved in ulceration and healing is essential for both patient and carer; the main reason why people with diabetes develop foot ulcers is the onset of sensory neuropathy which reduces the person's awareness of pressure, heat or trauma. The situation may be compounded by the characteristic clawing of the toes, resulting in additional pressure on the dorsum of the toes, the tips of the toes or under the head of the metatarsus bones. Many diabetic patients suffer from dryness of the skin due to autonomic neuropathy which increases the foot's susceptibility to trauma.

Diabetes is also associated with degenerative changes in blood vessels of all sizes [3]. Changes in the metatarsal arteries can result in obstruction by uniform thickening of the tunica intima, thereby severely restricting blood flow to the toes and giving rise to the development of tissue necrosis. Excessive callus formation also increases the risk of ulceration due to additional plantar pressure [4]. The Wagner classification system is widely used by chiropodists and diabetic nurse specialists to assess the severity of ulcers (Table 7.2).

Management priorities include regular removal of callus, control and prevention of infection using systemic antibiotics if appropriate, the relief of pressure which may be in the form of bed rest, crutches, felt pads, weight relieving casts, extra depth shoes or Besbock insoles. A recent study [5] suggests that the wearing of specially designed socks by people with highly insensitive feet will provide pressure relief

Table 7.2 Wagner classification scale

Grade One	Superficial ulcers at the site of high pressure
Grade Two	A deep ulcer that has arisen due to the continued destruction of the tissues leading to the involvement of underlying tendons
Grade Three	Further extension of the ulcer to involve bone, can develop osteomyelitis
Grade Four	Localized gangrene, commonly at ends of the toes and heels, may be associated with arterial insufficiency of the foot and can result in infective fasciitis
Grade Five	Extensive gangrene and tissue necrosis of the foot due usually to arterial occlusion

and offer an inexpensive addition to the methods currently available. Effective control of diabetes includes regular screening for complications such as neuropathy and retinopathy. Foot care education should emphasize especially the importance of daily examination of both feet, to include soles, dorsum and between the toes, the wearing of correctly fitting shoes, avoid walking barefoot and avoidance of thermal injuries, i.e. from hot water bottles. The shoes should be regularly inspected to ensure that there are no rough seams or edges or objects inside the shoes which may cause trauma to the tissues. Dressings should be provided that create an optimum local wound healing environment. If the patient does not respond to these measures then there is an exceedingly high risk of amputation.

MINOR BURNS

Burns result from dry heat and among the causes are flames, contact with hot surfaces, electric current and friction.

Scalds are produced by moist heat. Common causes are boiling water, tea and other beverages, hot fat and steam. For the purpose of this chapter, the term 'burn' will include injuries caused by scalding.

Burns are classified in severity according to two main factors [6]:

1. the body surface area burned (BSAB);
2. the depth of the burn.

BODY SURFACE AREA BURNED (BSAB)

This is, initially, the most crucial factor in determining the systemic effects of the injury and whether the patient will need resuscitation by means of intravenous infusion of fluid [7].

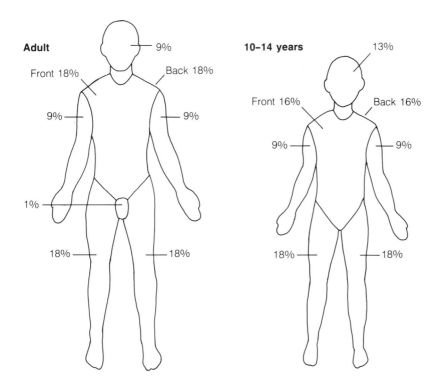

Figure 7.1 Wallace's Rule of Nines

Estimation of the BSAB is facilitated by the use of formulae such as Wallace's Rule of Nines (Figure 7.1) or by using dedicated charts, for example, the Lund and Browder Chart (Figure 7.2). A useful adjunct to these methods is the fact that the palmar surface of the patient's open hand with fingers together equals 1% of their body surface area. This is helpful when trying to estimate the percentage area of scattered burns, and may, for example, be used in conjunction with Wallace's Rule.

Children have differing body proportions from adults and the Lund and Browder charts are adaptable to take this into account. However, Wallace's Rule of Nines is only applicable to those patients over 14 years of age; an adapted version may be used for younger age groups (Figure 7.3).

When a burn injury occurs, the blood vessels in and around the injured area dilate and their walls develop increased permeability. Thus, fluid and proteins are lost from the circulation and there is venous stasis. Much of this fluid passes into the tissues, causing

Name_____ Ward_____ Number_____ Date_____

AGE_____ Admission weight_____

Lund and Browder charts

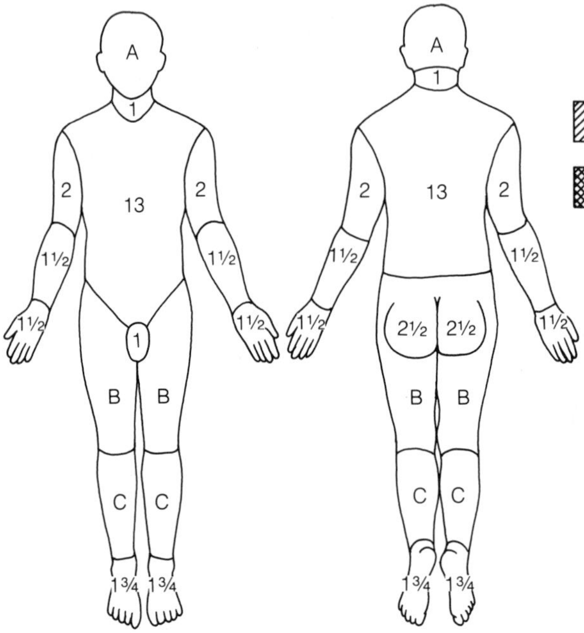

Ignore
simple erythema

Partial thickness loss
(PTL)

Full thickness loss
(FTL)

Region	PTL	FTL
Head		
Neck		
Ant. Trunk		
Post. Trunk		
Right arm		
Left arm		
Buttocks		
Genitalia		
Right leg		
Left leg		
Total burn·		

Relative percentage of body surface area
affected by growth

Area	Age 0	1	5	10	15	Adult
A = ½ of head	9½	8½	6½	5½	4½	3½
B = ½ of one thigh	2¾	3¼	4	4½	4½	4¾
C = ½ of one one leg	2½	2½	2¾	3	3¼	3½

Figure 7.2 Lund and Browder chart for estimating the severity of a burn wound.

Time of arrival		Inhalation injury present	Yes/no
Time of incident		Soot in throat/nose	Yes/no
First Aid given		Hoarse voice	Yes/no
		Intubation required	Yes/no
How long for		Size of tube	

| How accident happened |
| Clothing worn at time |
| Weight of patient |
| I.V. cannula size |
| Site of insertion |

Fluid regime (first four hours)

Hour	Fluid	Amount
1		
2		
3		
4		

Catheter passed	Yes/No
Catheter size	
Urine output	

Comments

Analgesia/antiemetics

Amount	Time

Tetanus toxoid (please tick)

Up to date ☐   Given ☐

Fluid regime

$$\frac{\text{Wt of pt} \times \text{\% of burn}}{2} = \text{Total fluids for infusion over next four hours.}$$

Figure 7.2 *continued*

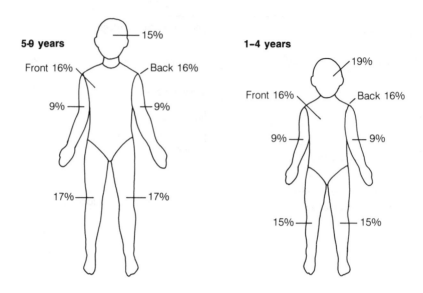

Figure 7.3 Wallace's Rule of Nines for children.

oedema. Some is lost from the surface of the skin as exudate or into the skin as blisters [8]. It can therefore be seen that the greater the area of burn, the greater the fluid loss and of course loss of excessive amounts of body fluid may cause hypovolaemic shock. Most of this fluid loss occurs within the first 48 hours of the burn and fortunately can be reasonably accurately forecast to allow for intravenous resuscitation regimes to be implemented if necessary [9]. This has allowed plastic surgeons to determine broad guidelines for the implementation of these intravenous resuscitation regimes. Where the size of the burn is greater than 15% of the body surface area in the adult, or 10% in the child, administration of intravenous fluids to combat shock is necessary [10]. These figures are merely guidelines and may be subject to adjustment according to the circumstances of the individual patient. Admission to hospital for such patients is of course essential. However, patients with much smaller percentage burns (who are able to combat fluid loss by oral administration of fluids) may still need to be admitted to hospital for other factors which arise from the burn injury (Table 7.3). Note that babies with burns of 5% or more of the body surface area should be admitted for resuscitation.

DEPTH OF BURN

The depth of the burn is also a critical factor to be considered when planning the clinical management of the burn injured patient.

Table 7.3 Inpatient management [8]

The following categories of patient require admission to hospital:

1. Adults with burns exceeding 15%, children with burns exceeding 10% and babies with burns exceeding 5% of the body surface.
2. Full thickness burns exceeding 1 in (2.5 cm) in diameter.
3. Full thickness burns of critical areas such as fingers and eyelids.
4. Burns which are circumferential round chest or a limb.
5. Burns of the face, hands, perineum, buttocks or feet.
6. Patients unable to be cared for adequately as outpatients.
7. Patients with potentially serious associated medical conditions, e.g. heart disease, other injuries.
8. Electrical burns.
9. Inhalation burns of hot or noxious gas or smoke.
10. Children whose injury is suspected of being non-accidental.

The assessment of burn depth [11] is largely subjective, being made by a combination of:

- the history of the injury;
- clinical observation
- sensation testing by pinprick.

Although there are guidelines for estimating the clinical depth of a burn (Figure 7.4), it is rare for a burn to be of completely uniform thickness. Indeed, experienced surgeons often initially encounter some difficulty in accurately predicting the depth of a burn [7].

Due to the major role the skin plays in helping to protect the body from harmful bacterial invasion, it can be seen that infection is a great threat to any burn injured patient, no matter how large or small the burn. Consequently, any handling of or contact with the wound must be undertaken with the highest standards of aseptic technique.

Providing infection is kept at bay, most superficial and partial thickness burns will heal satisfactorily within 7–14 days. This is because epithelium can quickly regenerate from the hair follicles, sweat ducts, etc. However, when the full thickness of the skin is destroyed (and indeed in some deeper partial thickness burns), not enough 'islands' capable of epithelial regeneration remain and the wound has to close by granulation. This is a slow process and produces a poor functional and cosmetic result, so these burns are best treated by skin grafting [12].

Therefore, any burn which does not heal within a maximum of three weeks following the injury should be considered for skin grafting; it is unnecessary to continue dressings for weeks after this time as skin grafting will heal the full thickness burn quickly [13]. Relatively small burns may thus need grafting if full thickness.

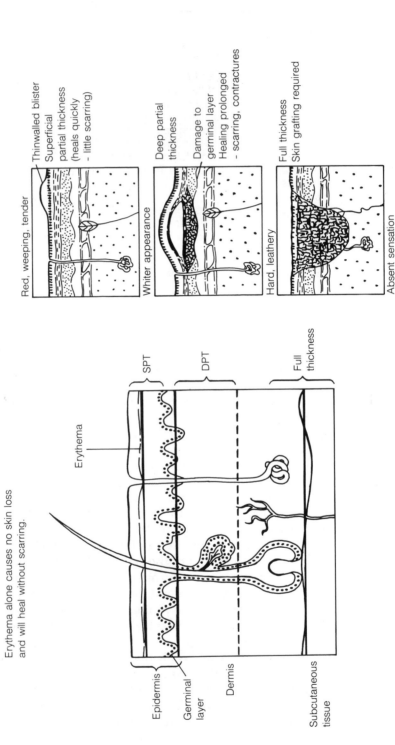

Figure 7.4 Depth of burn and clinical correlation.

NURSING MANGEMENT OF MINOR BURNS

Whether a burned patient is treated on an outpatient or inpatient basis is a decision which must be made by the medical staff. However, often the management of small burn wounds on an outpatient basis will be passed to the nursing staff, who assess and dress the wound as they deem appropriate (seeking medical opinion when necessary).

Some patients with minor burns (particularly children) may need to increase oral fluid intake for the first 48 hours following the injury and medical opinion must be sought in relation to the amount of fluid to be taken. It is usual to suggest that some salt be given along with the fluid to prevent water intoxication; in children, one of the proprietary mixtures used for water and electrolyte replacement in diarrhoea is suitable [9].

The patient's needs in respect of analgesia must be assessed on an individual basis and an appropriate analgesic may need to be prescribed by the medical staff. The effectiveness of analgesia should be monitored, with adjustments made as demanded by the patient's response. It is particularly important, especially for children, that adequate analgesic cover is given prior to dressing changes where difficulties are anticipated.

Although systemic antibiotics should not be given routinely for prophylaxis (in either major or minor burns) due to the risk of colonization with resistant organisms [10], the patient's tetanus immunization status should be ascertained. If not up-to-date, tetanus toxoid immunization should be given in line with the protocol for any open wound.

CARE OF THE MINOR BURN WOUND

Dressings

There is a bewildering array of dressings currently available which claim to be eminently suitable for use on minor burns. This is further complicated by restrictions of choice with regard to what is actually available for nursing staff to use in line with drug tariffs/hospital policies, etc. Therefore, rather than recommend specific products, it is better to consider the general principles which should be borne in mind when selecting a suitable dressing for a minor burn. According to Settle [10], the ideal burns dressing has the following properties:

- It should be absorbent enough to cope with potentially large amounts of exudate from the wound.
- It should be non-adherent, to avoid damaging delicate new epithelial cells on removal.
- The dressing should, as far as possible, act as a barrier to prevent outside bacteria penetrating to the wound surface.

In addition to Settle's recommendations, the dressing should also create the optimum conditions for re-epithelialization [14] and be capable of remaining *in situ* for 48–72 hours between dressing changes to avoid unnecessary disturbance of the delicate, newly growing epithelium [15].

As with any traumatic or surgical wound, a holistic approach to the problem must be taken. Alongside the choice of a suitable dressing, attention must be paid to those systemic factors which influence wound healing, such as the patient's nutritional status and underlying disease processes [16].

Dressing technique

There tends to be great local variation with regard to the treatment of the minor burn wound. Again, there can be no hard and fast rules to apply. For example, dealing with blisters remains a controversial area and various authors advocate differing approaches. Harvey-Kemble and Lamb [15] recommend complete debridement of all blisters and dead epithelium; Morgan and Wright [8] prefer to deroof and debride only large blisters, leaving the smaller ones intact; and Carson [13] favours the puncturing of blisters to let out the fluid, allowing the skin over the blister to fall back over the wound and so act as a form of 'biological dressing'. No objective evidence appears to exist to support any particular approach.

There are some principles, however, that appear to be common to most experts in this field and which therefore should be followed no matter what other variations in local practice exist. These are:

- maintenance of a scrupulous aseptic technique when performing these dressings;
- removal of any dirt and foreign material and cleansing of the wound prior to application of the first dressing;
- unless there are signs of infection or exudate 'strike-through' occurs, it is unnecessary to change the dressing more than 2–3 times per week;
- the burned area should be rested as much as possible until healed (e.g. with a sling for an arm burn);
- eschar (scab) should be gently removed with fine forceps and scissors, 7–10 days post injury;
- if a burn has not healed following a **maximum** of 21 days of conservative treatment, skin grafting should be considered without further delay [13].

BURNS OF SPECIAL AREAS

Eyelids

Burns involving the eyelids must be seen urgently by a plastic surgeon, as early skin grafting may be required. Chloramphenicol eye ointment may be applied to the area to prevent the eye drying out. Care must be taken with eyelids – if the lids are retracted, then an eyepad may cause corneal abrasions.

Face

Any burns to the face, other than those which are superficial and covering a small (i.e. less than 1% BSAB) area, should be referred for specialist opinion as soon as possible. The face does swell considerably when burned; patients need to be reassured that this is a normal reaction to injury and the swelling will start to subside in about 72 hours. Hospitalization of these patients is often necessary because of the danger of the swelling causing airway obstruction; there may also have been smoke inhalation and the patient will need to be monitored for signs of complications arising from this.

In hospital, facial burn wounds are most commonly treated by the semi-open method, applying a topical agent without dressings [15].

Hands

The backs of the hands are particularly vulnerable to deep burns, owing to the skin being relatively thin at this site. These burns heal slowly, which results in poor quality skin cover [10] and early skin grafting is therefore indicated.

Whilst burns of the palmar surface of the hands tend not to be so deep due to the greater thickness of skin, it is still recommended that all hand burns (other than very small superficial ones) should be referred for specialist opinion. The same protocol must apply to burns of the fingers; if mismanaged, the consequences for the patient can be catastrophic.

Hands swell considerably when burned and the affected hand(s) must be elevated as soon as practicable after the injury, in order to help minimize swelling. This elevation must continue during any journey to a specialist unit. The hands themselves may be temporarily dressed by enclosing them in a loose-fitting sterile plastic bag, lightly secured at the wrist with a bandage.

Electrical burns

The majority of electrical burns are due to contact with the domestic electrical supply and occur most commonly on the hands [7].

There is always an entry and an exit burn but they may differ greatly in severity [13].

Electricity follows the path of least resistance and therefore may follow blood vessels, nerves, etc. for some distance from the site of initial contact. Thus, electrical injury may often cause underlying damage to a much greater extent than would appear from the size of the skin burn. For this reason, it is recommended that all electrical injuries are thoroughly assessed by the medical staff.

This section has endeavoured to give a sufficient overview of the principles underpinning the physical management of the patient who has a 'minor' burn. More extensive information with regard to the care of burned patients can be obtained from some of the excellent texts used as references for this work.

MALIGNANT FUNGATING WOUNDS

Malignant fungating wounds are the visible markers of underlying malignant disease [17] and have a significant physical and psychological impact on a person's quality of life. The skin epithelium and its supporting blood and lymph vessels are infiltrated by a local tumour or metastatic cancerous cells. As the tumour enlarges it causes the capillary vessels to rupture with the subsequent development of tissue hypoxia and necrosis [18–20]. The lesions can appear as a raised fungating lesion or as an ulcerated crater with a distinct margin [21]. Breast lesions vary in size from a small encrusted area to an extensive malodorous and heavily exudating wound encompassing the chest wall and seen to be extending daily [22]. Neck and head lesions can be particularly challenging for both patient and carer because the effects of the disease and its treatment are highly visible and often stigmatizing [23].

Difficulty in finding suitable primary and secondary dressings and methods of fixation to meet the needs of the patient and the wound characteristics which allow the patient to socialize with confidence can also create further anxiety for both patient and carer [24]. The size and characteristics of the wound, such as the presence of necrotic tissue, excessive exudate production, malodour and bleeding, must all be assessed and documented [25] . It is essential that the nurse remains sensitive to the feelings and needs of both patient and immediate family and friends as the value of the nursing assessment is to some extent determined by the patient's ability or willingness

Table 7.4 Assessment of fungating lesions [22]

Level 1 Assessment

- Cause of wound
- Record of previous and current treatment
- General health status
- Body mass index* and nutritional intake
- Patient's environment and carer
- Socio-economic data
- Patient's and carer's insight into disease diagnosis and prognosis
- Patient's account of the impact of the wound on daily life
- Carer's account of the impact of the wound on daily life
- Health care support being provided

*May not be appropriate if patient has lymphoedema, oedema, ascites or is clearly cachectic

Wound assessment

What is the form of the wound?
- Ulcerating
- Hidden extensions
- Tissue type
- Black/brown necrotic tissue
- Yellow slough
- Exudate low/moderate/copious
- Odour
- Bleeding
- Fistula
- Type of fistula fluid
- Wound contaminated
- Wound clinically infected, bacterial or fungal
- Is there any pain and/or pruritus?

What is the condition of the surrounding skin?
- Nodular
- Fragile
- Sensitive
- Adherent/non-adherent
- Macerated
- Dry, unbroken
- Moist desquamation

Wound site and size
- Describe the wound location
- Is the wound's surface flat or curved?
- What is the surface area?
- What is the height of nodules?
- What is the depth of ulcer?

Outcome of Level 1 assessment

Information gained from the wound assessment will indicate:
- wound pathology, treatment and progression
- patient's and carer's knowledge and acceptance of diagnosis/prognosis
- emotional impact of wound

Table 7.4 *cont'd*

- social impact of wound
- patient's environment, ability to self-care and informal support systems
- level of formal health care systems
- data on the form, site and accompanying symptoms of the wound

Level 2 Assessment

Application of critical thinking skills:
- Are the treatment options, i.e. surgery, radiotherapy, chemotherapy, hormone therapy, exhausted?
- Can the patient's prognosis be estimated in days, weeks or months? Does this influence wound management?
- What are the patient's priorities? What are the carer's priorities? Are they realistic? Do they differ? Do they differ from the multidisciplinary team view?
- What resources do the patient and carer have to meet their priorities?
- What level and aspect of multidisciplinary team support is appropriate for the patient and carer?
- What multidisciplinary team support is available?

Outcome of Level 2 Assessment

The assessment should provide:
- a statement of symptom control needs in relation to the wound
- an insight into patient, carer and multidisciplinary team priorities for wound care
- reconciliation of any differences in these priorities

1. What professional interventions are needed for wound management? The following factors need to be considered in relation to individual symptom control needs:

- Debridement of necrotic tissue
- Control of bacterial/fungal infection
- Control of exudate
- Control of odour
- Anticipation and modification of complications, such as bleeding
- Pain control
- Minimal disturbance to the patient from dressing changes
- Dressing removal without trauma
- Cosmetic acceptability
- Stoma care products for fistula management
- Care of skin surrounding the lesion

2. Criteria for selection of dressing products:

- The wound is debrided to remove excess exudate and toxic materials, to prevent deterioration and control smell.
- The dressing is removed without trauma because the interface between the dressing and the wound is exudate.
- Pain control is achieved through maintenance of optimum humidity at the wound site.
- Dressings used can be left *in situ* for one to five days.
- Cosmetic acceptability must be considered and primary dressings should be used, where possible, instead of bulky dressings.

Table 7.4 *cont'd*

Other points to consider include:
● Will dressing materials, based on moist wound healing theory, meet the patient's symptom control needs?
● Can conditions at the wound site support extended periods between dressing changes, i.e. beyond 24 hours?
● Who should do the dressing changes, patient, carer or nurse?
● Are the choices made cost-effective in terms of money and time and are they available?

3. Consider with the multidisciplinary team the need for adjuvant therapies for the control of:
● bleeding from tumour with antifibrinolytics/haemostats
● odour due to aerobic/anaerobic colonization with topical metronidazole
● odour from organic materials (e.g. putrescine/cadavarine) during wound debridement with charcoal dressings
● pain with analgesics/corticosteroids/tricyclics
● pruritus with corticosteroids

4. Is specialist input, such as social worker or palliative care support team, required?

5. Which environment will provide the most appropriate support for the patient and carer - home, hospice, hospital?

6. What is available in the patient's locality?

to communicate, given the great lengths some patients of all ages go to to conceal their condition from even those closest to them. The nurse's own communication skills and the application of critical thinking skills are the key to effective patient dialogue. A framework using a problem solving approach is offered in Table 7.4.

If the management of a fungating lesion is to be effective it must be based on close collaboration between the multidisciplinary team and patient, it is only when treatment options are exhausted that the emphasis of the team shifts from cure or long term control to the palliation of symptoms [26]. The dynamic nature of these lesions provides a constant challenge to the practitioner compounded by a dearth of research based knowledge upon which to base one's decisions. An example of different treatment options that have been used by practitioners with varying degrees of success are offered in Table 7.5.

Consideration must also be given to the patient care environment; is the patient at home, in hospital or a hospice? This may be the key factor in determining which dressings can be used as the limitations imposed by the drug tariff greatly reduces user choice. Wherever possible the dressing should be acceptable to the patient as well as meeting the requirements of their wound and lifestyle. Some patients prefer to care for the wound themselves or with the help of a family

Table 7.5 Treatment options

Radiotherapy	Reduces the size of the tumours, not suitable for patients with radiation induced tumours or who are unable to tolerate further treatments
Chemotherapy	Usually used in palliation treatment, can be associated with a low response rate and unpleasant side effects. Patients given low dose combination therapy have fewer side effects
Hormonal therapy	Altering the hormonal environment may reduce the size and progression of the tumour
Wound cleansing	Removal of debris by gentle irrigation, bathing or showering reduces the risk of infection. Water or sodium chloride 0.9% are the solutions of choice as antiseptics are quickly inactivated by wound debris. Some patients may experience discomfort or pain when the wound is cleansed
Debridement of necrotic tissue	Debridement will treat or reduce the risk of infection, malodour and excessive exudate. Surgical removal is rapid but this technique is only suitable for the minority of patients. Suitable alternatives to rehydrate and remove necrotic tissue and slough are amorphous gels, polysaccharide beads, alginate dressings or hydrocolloids
Control of bleeding	The haemostat properties of alginate dressings are especially valuable in the control of bleeding. Occasionally it may be necessary to cauterize leaking vessels or use oral antifibrinolytic agents as prescribed.
Control of malodour	Debridement of necrotic tissue, especially if combined with the use of topical metronidazole, has been demonstrated to be an effective method of odour control. The application of an activated charcoal dressing can also be of value
Control of excessive exudate	Hydrogels, alginate and polyurethane foam dressings are all suitable options for the management of excessive exudate (see Chapter 4)

member/friend or may share the management with the professional carers, a fact also to be considered when deciding on treatment options.

Although the precise incidence of fungating lesions is unknown, as data are estimated rather than derived from population based cancer registers [27], the impact on the individual's lifestyle can be devastating. There are many questions that still need to be asked and answers sought about the management of fungating lesions.

RADIATION DAMAGED SKIN

The use and effects of radiotherapy to treat some malignant tumours are well recognized and documented [28–36]. Continuing advancement within this field of technology now enables much deeper tumours to be treated with greater precision [37], thereby reducing the effects of radiation damage to the surrounding skin. The onset of any adverse reaction usually manifests within seven days following the commencement of treatment and is of limited duration. The effects, however, can be extremely unpleasant for the patient whose quality of life may already be compromised by the presence of the tumour.

Radiation affects the basal cells in the skin epidermis which are constantly dividing, making them extremely sensitive to this form of treatment and hence more susceptible to an adverse reaction. Damaged epithelium manifests as a generalized mild or marked area of erythema due to vasodilatation of the underlying capillaries. The patient may also complain of localized itching and irritation followed by the development of dry scaling desquamation as the damaged cells deslough. If the tissue damage is more severe the skin may blister and present as moist desquamation associated with deeper tissue loss and a statistically significant increased risk of developing telangiectasis [30] or fibrosis. The precise incidence and severity of radiation damage is unknown as no national data are available.

PREVENTION AND TREATMENT

The current dearth of research based papers on the prevention and treatment of radiation damaged skin has led to a wide variety of products and techniques being used, some based upon sound logical principles, others unproven and of questionable value which should probably be discontinued [38]. The risk of damage may be reduced by eliminating as far as possible anything that causes friction to the at-risk areas, such as bathing, thus avoiding the need to disturb the vulnerable tissue. If this is not an acceptable option the patient should be advised to avoid the use of perfumed soaps, talcum powder or lotions and to be especially careful not to damage the skin by friction when drying the area. The use of baby oil appears an acceptable alternative as a soothing lotion. More recently, the use of a homoeopathic cream has been advocated [39], although the original findings (1989) were based on a sample population of 20 patients. Further assessment of this product continues to support its use [40].

A multicentre study was undertaken [41] involving 300 patients who, following mastectomy or lumpectomy for breast cancer, were subsequently referred for radiotherapy. The purpose of the study was to see if dietary fatty acid supplements protect patients against radiation induced injury of the skin as assessed by measuring erythema.

Pain and tissue damage can be exacerbated by inappropriate wound and skin care. Table 7.5 offers treatment options based on empirical evidence.

REFERENCES

1. Tovey, F.E. (1984) The manufacture of diabetic footwear. *Diabetic Med*, 1, 69–71.
2. Mallins, J.M. (1968) *Clinical Diabetes Mellitus*, Eyre and Spottiswoode, London.
3. Wagner, F.W. (1981) The dysvascular foot: a system for diagnosis and treatment. *Foot Ankle*, 2–64.
4. Fletcher, E. (1992) Foot problems in people with diabetes. *Nursing Standard*, 6(37), 25–8.
5. Murray, H.J., Veves, A., Young, M.J., Richie, D.H. and Boulton, A.J. (1993) Role of experimental socks in the foot care of the high risk diabetic foot. A multicentre patient evaluation study of experimental hosiery in the diabetic foot. *Diabetes Care*,18(8), 1190–2.
6. Harvey-Kemble, J.V. and Lamb, B.E. (1987) *Practical Burns Management*, Hodder and Stoughton, London.
7. Muir, I.F.K., Barclay, T.L. and Settle, J.A.D. (1986) *Burns and Their Treatment*, 3rd edn, Butterworth, London.
8. Morgan, B. and Wright, M. (1986) *Essentials of Plastic and Reconstructive Surgery*, Faber and Faber, London.
9. Wilmshurst, A.M. (1991) Resuscitation of the burnt patient. *Salisbury Med J*, 80, 786–90.
10. Settle, J.A.D. (1986) *Burns – The First Five Days*, Smith and Nephew, Romford.
11. Rossi, L.F.A. and Shakespeare, P.G. (1991) Surgical management of burn injuries. *Salisbury Med J*, 80, 797–810.
12. Shakespeare, P.G. (1991) Cultured human skin epithelium for burn wound repair. *Salisbury Med J*, 80, 820–7.
13. Cason, J.S. (1981) *Treatment of Burns*, Chapman & Hall, London.
14. Dealey, C. (1991) Criteria for wound healing. *Nursing*, 4(29), 20–1.
15. Harvey-Kemble, J.V. and Lamb, B.E. (1984) *Plastic Surgical and Burns Nursing*, Baillière Tindall, London.
16. Spencer, K.E. and Bale, S. (1990) A logical approach (management of surgical wounds). *Prof Nurse*, 5, 303–8.
17. Rutherford, M. and Foxley, D. (1990) Awareness of psychological needs, in *Palliative Care for People with Cancer*, (eds J. Penson and R. Fisher), Edward Arnold, London.
18. Sims, R. and Fitzgerald, V. (1985) *Community Nursing Management of Patients with Ulcerating Malignant Breast Disease*, RCN/Oncology Nursing Society, London.

19. Thomas, S. (1992) *Current Practices in the Management of Fungating Lesions and Radiation Damaged Skin*, Surgical Materials Testing Laboratory, Bridgend.
20. Moody, M. and Grocott, P. (1993) Let us extend our knowledge base: assessment and management of fungating malignant wounds. *Prof Nurse*, **8**(9), 586–90.
21. Grocott, P. and Moody, M. (1993) *A Practical Approach to the Management of Malignant Fungating Wounds*, booklet published for study day organized by *Professional Nurse*, available from the authors.
22. Fairbairn, K. (1993) Towards better care for women. *Prof Nurse*, **9**(3), 204–12.
23. Blackmore, S. (1988) Body image: the oncological perspective, in *Altered Body Image. The Nurse's Role*, (ed. M. Salter), John Wiley and Sons, Chichester.
24. Collinson, G.P. (1993) Fungating malignant wounds. II Nursing management. *Wound Man*, **4**(2), S4–S5.
25. Bale, S. (1993) *Cavity Wounds*, educational leaflet No. 11, Wound Care Society.
26. Banks, V. and Jones, V. (1993) Palliative care of a patient with terminal nasal carcinoma. *J Wound Care*, **2**(1), 14–15.
27. Grocott, P. (1993) Fungating malignant wounds. I An overview and priorities for palliative management. *Wound Man*,**4**(2), S2–S3.
28. Arimoto, T., Maruhashi, N. *et al.* (1989) Acute skin reactions observed in fractionated proton irradiation. *J Rad Med*, **7**(1),23–7.
29. Bentzen, S.M., Thames, H.D. and Overgaard, M. (1989) Latent-time estimation for late cutaneous and subcutaneous radiation reaction in a single follow-up clinical study. *J Radiother Oncol*, **15**(3), 267–74.
30. Bentzen, S.M. and Overgaard, M. (1991) Relationship between early and late normal-tissue injury after post mastectomy radiotherapy. *J. Radiother Oncol*, **20**(3) 159–65.
31. Husband, J.D., Errington, R.D. *et al.* (1992) Accelerated fast neutron therapy: a pilot study.*Br J. Radiol*, **65** (776), 691–6.
32. Shirato, H., Gupta, N.K., Jordan, T.J. and Hendry, J.H. (1990) Lack of late skin necrosis in man after high dose irradiation using small field sizes: experiences of grid therapy. *Br J Radiol*, **63**(775), 871.
33. Turesson, I. and Thames, H.D. (1989) Repair capacity and kinetics of human skin during fractionated radiotherapy: erythema, desquamation and telangiectasia after 3 and 5 years follow-up. *J Radiother Oncol*, **15**(2), 169–88.
34. Van Limbergen, E., Briot, E. and Orijkoningen, N. (1990) The source–skin distance, measuring bridge: a method to avoid radiation telangiectasia in the skin after interstitial therapy for breast cancer. *Int J Radiat Oncol, Biol, Phys*, **18**(5), 1239–44.
35. Van der Schueren, E., Vanden Bogaert, W. *et al.* (1990) Radiotherapy by multiple fractions per day (MFD) in head and neck cancer: acute reactions of skin and mucosa. *Int J Radiat Oncol, Biol, Phys*, **19**(2), 301–11.
36. Varga, J., Haustein, U.F. *et al.* (1991) Exaggerated radiation induced fibrosis in patients with systemic sclerosis. *JAMA*, **265**(24), 3292–5.
37. Moody, M. (1993) Radiation damaged skin: which treatment option and why? *Wound Man*, **4**(4), 56–7.

38. Thomas, S. (1992) *Current Practices in the Management of Fungating Lesions and Radiation Damaged Skin*, Surgical Materials Testing Laboratory, Bridgend.
39. Lawton, J. and Twomey, J. (1990) *Skin Reactions to Radiotherapy for Breast Cancer, A Report for Health Professionals Involved in the Care of Women with Breast Cancer*, Calderdale Health Authority.
40. Lawton, J. (1993) Personal correspondence.
41. Jackson, B. (1993) Can oral fatty acid supplements moderate radiation reactions? *Wound Man*, **4**(2), 57.

FURTHER READING

WOUND DEHISCENCE, FISTULA AND SINUS FORMATION

Borwell, B. (1994) Nursing management of the patient with a gastro-intestinal fistula. *J. Tissue Viability*, **4**(1), 23–6.
Everett, W.G. (1985) Wound sinus and fistula, in *Wound Care*, (ed. S. Westaby), Heinemann Medical, London.
Moorehead, R.J. (1992) *The Emergency Management of Wounds*. Proceedings of 1st European Conference on Advances in Wound Management, (ed. K. Harding), Macmillan, Basingstoke.
Perkins, P. (1992) Wound dehiscence: causes and care. *Nursing Standard*, **6**(34), 12–14.
Westaby, S. (1985) *Wound Care*, Heinemann Medical, London.

DIABETIC FOOT ULCERATION

Barnett, A. and Odugbesan, O. (1987) Foot care for diabetics. *Nursing Times*, **83**(2), 24–6.
Bloom, A. and Ireland, J. (1992) *A Colour Atlas of Diabetes*, 2nd edn, Wolfe Medical, London.
Conor, H., Boulton, A.J.M. and Ward, J.D. (1987) *The Foot in Diabetes*, John Wiley and Sons, Chichester.
Elkeleles, R.S. and Wolfe, J.H.N. (1991) ABC of vascular disease. The diabetic foot. *Br Med J*, **199**(303), 1053–5.
Fanis, I. (1992) *The Management of the Diabetic Foot*, 2nd edn, Churchill Livingstone, London.
Jones, G.R. (1991) Walking casts: effective treatment for foot ulcers. *Pract Diabetes*, **8**(4), 131–6.
Thurston, R. and Beattie, C. (1984) Foot lesions in diabetics: care of a patient. *Nursing Times*, **80**, 48–50.
Young, M. (1993) *Blueprint for the Management of Diabetic Foot Ulceration*, ConvaTec Ltd, Harrington House, Milton Road, Uxbridge.
Young, M. and Boulton, A.J. M. (1991) Guidelines for identifying the at-risk foot. *Pract Diabetes*, **8**(3), 103–5.

Specialist wound care units

8

Previous chapters have emphasized how common wound care problems are in both hospital and community populations yet few people are fortunate enough to gain access to expert advice. The majority of wound care opinions are given by nurses who have gained their own experience or have been motivated to seek specialist tuition. A few have become wound care specialist nurses or tissue viability nurses who disseminate their knowledge by teaching others in addition to having a clinical workload. Doctors with a specialist interest in wounds are even more rare. Specialists include dermatologists, diabetologists, physicians in care of the elderly, vascular surgeons, rheumatologists, rehabilitation physicians and bioengineers. Other specialists have become involved (in small numbers) and these include occupational therapists, podiatrists, pharmacists and dietitians, though this is obviously not an exhaustive list.

Shared problems and the sense of the subject being somewhat a 'Cinderella' have led to the formation of numerous groups and societies whose aims include increased awareness of the problem of chronic wounds, more medical and lay education, more research and better clinical care, the Wound Care Society and the Tissue Viability Society being just two. These and others run local study days, regional, national and European conferences. Their combined membership runs into thousands and their combined audiences via books, newsletters, articles, study days and conferences must be tens of thousands. Yet go into any district general hospital and every teaching hospital and within minutes you will find the signs to the coronary care unit and its supporting cardiology department. Try to find the equivalent wound care unit. You will do so at the University Hospital of Wales, Cardiff (under the directorship of Dr Keith Harding), at Odstock Hospital in Salisbury, the Royal London Hospital (Mile End) and of course Stoke Mandeville Hospital. There are a few others yet it is one of the anomalies of the National Health Service that necrosis of a tiny amount of cardiac tissue (with admittedly life-threatening complications) has engendered hundreds of specialist units whereas necrosis of massive amounts of tissue (with less immediate but nonetheless life-threatening consequences) generates wound care units that can be counted on the fingers of both hands.

The situation is beginning to change, however. The government is becoming interested in the mammoth cost to the NHS of chronic wounds in its ever continuing quest for value for money. Health care workers themselves are getting together within both hospital and community settings and identifying areas of mutual interest which in addition have benefit to patients, purchasers and providers, e.g. (incidence and prevalence data, comparisons of dressings costs and the use of wound formularies to save money, more effective treatment regimes – in the field of venous ulceration, the Riverside multi-layer bandaging technique, etc.).

Key people in these local initiatives have been the specialist wound care nurses. The next stage should be a consolidation of these achievements and a broadening of impact by developing multidisciplinary wound care groups. These groups need to have access to a range of expertise either as core members or as coopted or available help. Advice will be needed from pharmacists, dietitians, statisticians, hospital management, clinicians, specialist and community nurses, general practitioners and many others. This group will need to advise hospital trusts, community trusts, GP fundholders and district health authorities and liaise frequently with purchasers and providers. The issues will involve data gathering concerning chronic wounds (now included in many contracts), pressure sore prevention advice to hospital clinicians, hospital nurses and all other relevant groups, presentations and reports to management to identify savings in product usage that can be channelled into direct patient care via prevention and treatment techniques.

In many districts, once this group has been set up, identified the issues and begun tackling them, it is a natural extension into the development of a resource centre/education and research facility/ clinical management base, i.e. a wound care unit. In the US wound care units are numerous and have been developed over many years. There are many models and the health service system there obviously leads to some incompatible features. The basic guidelines concerning what to think about when contemplating such a unit, however, are very similar and as our health service system tries increasingly to emulate that in the US, the incompatibilities get fewer by the day –profit supplanting the excellence of patient care.

The issues involved in setting up a wound care clinic were the subject of a postconference workshop of the Advanced Wound Care

Symposium held in San Diego, California, in April 1993. Distinguished US experts in wound care, including Evonne Fowler and Gerit Mulder, shared their experiences at that workshop and outlined the business plan guidelines needed [1].

BUSINESS PLAN GUIDELINES

SETTING THE STRATEGIC DIRECTION

1. Mission statement (a global statement that provides a shared sense of purpose, direction and achievement).

   This is best arrived at by the multidisciplinary team conducting a SWOT (strengths, weaknesses, opportunities and threats) exercise. This is a management tool that encourages participation and identifies pertinent issues for the individuals concerned early on. A cohesive approach is fostered and from all the issues identified, a statement is arrived at that encompasses the ideals of the project participants.
2. Long term goals (3–5 years).
3. Short term objectives and indicators (one year).
4. Strategies (how you are going to accomplish the objectives):
   - What service are you going to provide?
   - How will you reduce costs for your institution?
   - How will you market the services?
   - Will establishing a clinic require internal reorganization (staffing changes, reporting and admitting mechanisms, coordination with other disciplines, etc.)?
   - How often are you going to review the programme to measure progress (quarterly reviews are recommended)?

MARKET RESEARCH AND ANALYSIS

1. Start-up costs (possible lease or inter-service agreement, renovation of space, staffing, equipment, start-up supplies, etc.).
2. Expected revenues (based on projected number of referrals – either part of existing contracts, tertiary referrals or extracontractual ECR, charges per follow-up visit/outpatient attendance, clinical trials, etc.).
3. General expenses (staffing, utilities, repair and maintenance, office supplies, postage, photocopying, patient supplies, etc.).
4. Net income projection (whatever sources) versus total expenditure on unit.

The separate issues can be looked at more closely to build up a picture of the potential unit, be it simple or complex.

STAFFING

- Medical – day to day junior/senior medical cover, rotas, sick cover, study leave, etc. Access to specialist opinions.
- Nursing – junior/senior staffing, role of clinical nurse specialist, night duty, rotas, etc.
- Research – both medical and nursing. Clinical trial work, allied to other research units, e.g. experimental dermatology, bioengineering, surgical.
- Administration – admissions, ward clerk, transport, coordinating discharges, filing, etc.
- Management – strategic view, budgets, contracts, etc.

SERVICES

- Clinical
- Research
- Education/teaching – local community hospital staff/community staff
  - customized courses in wound healing (on and off site)
  - undergraduate medical/nursing
  - postgraduate medical/nursing
- Referral/consulting service – hospital and community
- Clinical monitoring/standard setting
- Animal studies (approved specialist centres only)

PREREQUISITES

- Facility
- Staffing – minimum per bed ratio for nurses, medical, administrative, paramedical support, cost effective ratio beds/staffing/space/rotas.
- Equipment – non-invasive vascular testing
  - debridement
  - wound care products
  - instrument sterilization facilities/access
  - research (refrigerators/incubators)
- Access – multidisciplinary team members
  - emergency specialist teams
  - laboratory facilities
  - radiology
  - physical therapy
  - social worker/community social work teams

CLINICAL MANAGEMENT INITIATIVES

- Preadmission screening
- Decrease length of stay
- Consistent continuity of care
- Increased quality of care
- Self-development
- Staff development
- Cost effective care
- Time effective management
- Local wound care
- Self-care teaching
- Carers' wound care teaching
- Monitor/management/compliance

SHOWING EFFECTIVENESS/QUALITY ASSURANCE

- Readmission rate
- Nurse visits
- Referrals to district nurses
- Complete healing rates
- Improvement rates
- Satisfaction surveys (physicians/staff/patients)

TOTAL QUALITY MANAGEMENT

- Training
- Case management
- Database monitoring
- Quality assurance
- Management

PRODUCTS

- Diverse
- Not favouring a single product/company
- Appropriate product selection
- Wound care formulary
- Research based product change

MARKETING

- In-service programme
- Community activities

- Printed materials
- Study days
- Conferences

MANAGEMENT MODELS

There are various management models for wound care units. In the US the hospital based, nurse managed model is the most common.

- Referring doctor
- Progress report
- Dietary advice ← nurse specialist → diabetes advice
- Panel of specialist consultants

In the UK it is to be hoped that many different management models will be created depending on the local circumstances. I would anticipate the emergence of the physician or physician/nurse management model as the two most likely UK models.

WOUND CARE UNIT DATABASE (INFORMATION TECHNOLOGY)

- General client data
- Wound summary
- Treatment summary
- Outcome report
- Quality assurance report

Each wound care unit will need to develop its own wound management protocol. Each component of the protocol can be expanded in the clinical setting and most clinics devise a proforma which provides a record of all the data needed and also acts as an aide memoire for the personnel involved. The proformas usually include detailed personal history (often in the form of a checklist so that specific data can be extracted later), for example:

- mental status
- activity level
- body type
- nutritional
- incontinence
- sleep pattern.

A detailed past medical history checklist is included with specific questions concerning diagnostic and treatment procedures as well as all prescription and over-the-counter medication. The patient gives a brief history of the specific wound and any illness and a wound documentation record is filled out, usually including the following categories:

- type
- stage
- location
- size
- depth of wound bed
- colour
- exudate
- odour
- surrounding skin condition
- photographic results
- culture results
- biochemical results.

A wound management checklist ensures that some essential issues are not overlooked:

- Doppler examination
- pain chart
- diabetes exluded
- patient education plan formulated and explained.

Wound product selection may also be organized by means of a checklist if required. The principles of wound management have already been covered in Chapter 4.

The following wound management protocol was developed at the Kaiser Bellflower Medical Center, California, and used as a teaching example at the postconference symposium on Wound Care Clinics: State of the Art, in San Diego, California, April 1993.

PURPOSE

- Differentiate wound by classification
- Identify/address/correct underlying cause(s) of wound(s)
- Use appropriate treatment in cost effective manner
- Prevent complications: infections/amputation

ASSESSMENT

- History – clinical examination
- Laboratory studies: culture/sensitivity/biopsy
- Nutritional history
- Cardiovascular status
- Diabetes status

- Wound profile
  - Description
  - Measurements
  - Photography
- Non-invasive vascular testing
  - BP
  - Pulses: dorsalis pedis/posterior tibial
  - Doppler
  - Doppler wave form testing
  - Ankle/arm Doppler pressure index
  - $TcPO_2$ (transcutaneous oxygen tension analysis)
- Invasive vascular testing
  - Consultant vascular opinion
  - Arteriogram
  - Proximal balloon occlusive inflow arteriography and digital arteriography
- Radiology testing
  - X-ray
  - Wound present longer than four weeks – determine presence of osteomyelitis
- If X-ray changes are subtle or suspicious of osteomyelitis:
  - bone scan
  - bone biopsy
  - bone culture

DIFFERENTIAL DIAGNOSIS

- Trauma
- Postoperative wound complication
- Pressure ulcers
- Collagen disease
- Burns
- Arterial ulcers
- Venous ulcers
- Diabetic ulcers

INTERVENTIONS

- Local wound care
  - Cleansing
  - Debridement
  - Covering
- Infection control
- General measures

- Pressure reduction/relief/offloading
- Nutrition
- Exercise
- Stop smoking
- Pain control
- Medication
- Compression therapy
  - Control oedema
  - Elevation
  - Support stockings
  - Compression bandage
  - Sequential compression device
- Other measures
  - Growth factor therapy
  - Tissue extender
  - Diapulse
  - Ultrasound
  - Electrical stimulation
  - Hydrosound
- Surgical intervention
  - Vascular reconstruction
  - Grafts
- Orthotics
  - Footwear examined/recommendations made
  - Relieve pressure points
  - Stretching the shoe
- Temporary cut-out areas to relieve pressure
  - Placement of metatarsal
  - Plastizote inserts

PATIENT TEACHING

- Early intervention
- Wound care
- Prevention of complications
- Nutritional requirements
- Stop smoking
- Exercise
- Foot care
- Regular check-ups

The above protocol can provide a template or baseline for each unit to modify individually according to local requirements. The protocols, however, provide a uniformity of approach which becomes vital in the areas of quality assurance, data collection and research.

As we approach the 21st century the clinical, financial and political health imperatives will result in wound care achieving major significance. To achieve a holistic approach with clinical excellence, research and education as the three base points, wound care units must become available to all patients who require their multi-disciplinary expertise. The amateur climate of wound care has passed, the professional one is upon us bringing with it exacting standards and clinical challenges. These units must become centres of excellence in all their components – clinical management, research and education. The next generation of doctors and nurses must receive tuition in the subject of wound care at an undergraduate level to equip them with the knowledge base needed to manage patients properly. Part of this training can be based at these centres as their numbers expand.

'Would you tell me please, which way I ought to go from here?' asked Alice.
'That depends a good deal on where you want to get to,' said the cat.
'I don't much care where,' said Alice.
'Then it doesn't matter which way you go,' said the cat.
Lewis Carroll, *Alice's Adventures in Wonderland*

REFERENCES

1. Kotler, P. and Clarke, R.N. (1987) *Marketing for Healthcare Organisations*, Prentice-Hall Inc., New Jersey.

Education and legal issues

9

MEDICAL EDUCATION

The current concept that wound care is a multidisciplinary science/art has a major weakness. The medical input (with a few notable exceptions) is usually woefully inadequate. The majority of doctors do not possess the communication skills, the wound care language, to be full partners in the assessment and treatment procedures. Other professional groups have recognized this training deficiency, responded with appropriate education packages and thus truly joined the team, e.g. dietitians/nutritionists, pharmacists. Medical undergraduates have been less fortunate in this training process. From the day they qualify the junior doctor's main responsibility is the acquisition of appropriate information concerning the patient, a comprehensive examination including every organ system and the setting out of a basic management and, if necessary, prevention plan to be agreed with more senior colleagues. There is necessary and invaluable communication with the nursing staff responsible for that patient at almost every stage.

It is therefore perplexing to consider the plight of a junior doctor when confronted with a patient who has a chronic wound (e.g. leg ulcer) or acutely developing wound (e.g. pressure sore) as part of or even as their main medical condition. Most medical undergraduates do not know the aetiological factors behind the formation of chronic wounds, do not know how to assess a wound accurately and do not know the rudiments of basic management or prevention. In addition they cannot usefully discuss this part of the patient's condition with the nursing staff to whom responsibility for assessment, management and prevention has been completely delegated.

This state of affairs may have persisted for a lot longer were it not for the emergence of litigation episodes. When things were perceived to go wrong the full force of the legal profession was seen to fall on the one group of staff who had no choice but to care for the patient – the nurses. Regularly the nursing staff were not supported by their medical colleagues and they rightly felt scapegoated. The consultant in charge of the patient takes overall responsibility for all other aspects of care and this area should be no different (barring obvious negligence on the part of a team member). The management of an at-risk client is a team affair with various members of the team taking lead responsibility at different times. Early on in the admission the medical/nursing interface is crucial. Assessment and communication may indicate, for instance, that a client has been on the floor for many hours and that pressure damage has already occurred. The management plan includes trying to prevent any further damage but also discussion with client and family explaining the situation so that later there is no misunderstanding as to the cause of the damage.

What is the evidence for this disastrous state of affairs?

In 1991 I undertook a survey with the help of the Tissue Viability Society [1]. A brief postal questionnaire was sent to the Deans of all 27 medical schools and colleges in England, Scotland, Wales and Northern Ireland. The Deans were requested to circulate copies of the questionnaire to all departments involved in the teaching on chronic wounds (excluding the teaching of basic pathology and histology of wounds). The questionnaire was computer coded on completion and return rendered anonymous.

There were 19 replies (a 70% response rate). Two medical schools/colleges indicated that there was definitely no formal teaching and four thought that there was 'probably' no teaching. The average amount of teaching was six hours (range 0–35.5 hours). There were marked regional variations with England and Wales (excluding London) averaging less than two hours teaching, London six hours and Scotland 17 hours.

Two thirds of respondents indicated that all the students received the teaching whereas one third showed that only specific 'firms' or groups of students received the tuition. The teaching took place predominantly in the first clinical year. The list of teachers is shown in Table 9.1.

The total numbers indicate that some students get teaching from more than one specialty though Dermatology, Health Care of the Elderly and, perhaps surprisingly, General Surgery feature most.

Seventy percent of students have some form of examination on the material taught but only 59% have this work examined in the final MB or in continuous assessment examinations. Concerning the content of the material taught, 81% of teachers included preventative aspects, 62% the use of pressure relieving equipment and aids, 81% the use of various wound dressings but only 50% included any elementary bioengineering or its application, i.e. physiological measurement.

Table 9.1 Who teaches the subject?

• Dermatology	11
• Health Care of the Elderly	7
• General Medicine	2
• General Surgery	7
• Vascular Surgery	3
• Plastic Surgery	4
• Orthopoedic Surgery	3
• Accident and Emergency	1
• Chiropody	1
• Nursing	1

The survey highlights the lamentable lack of education concerning the prevention and management of chronic open wounds that most of our medical undergraduates are receiving. Some questionnaires were returned with detailed letters of explanation outlining the reasons behind the paucity of appropriate teaching. These ranged from the honest – 'In simple truth there is no structured teaching whatsoever on the management of wounds' – through the informative – 'The General Medical Council will be issuing new guidelines about the medical curriculum late this year'– to the frankly pompous – 'the business of a medical school into the 1990s is learning rather than teaching ... we do not think this task is about stuffing them with even more provision (data) for the journey: their canoe will sink'.

Using the same analogy, medical students should be taught to swim and life-save as there is less danger of their canoe sinking than the patient drowning. Chronic open wounds may be an unglamorous aspect of medical life, they affect particularly the elderly and especially the elderly sick, yet the resultant morbidity and mortality is considerable. Cost issues apart, doctors must intellectually and morally join the other specialties dealing with these patients. This will not happen unless the management of chronic open wounds becomes a compulsory addition to the medical undergraduate curriculum and as such is examined in the final MB. There is currently and for the foreseeable future no shortage of patients.

Further research into medical awareness was carried out in the University Teaching Hospital in Manchester [2]. A pressure sore awareness survey was conducted in a 800-bed teaching hospital. A confidential semistructured questionnaire was used after an initial pilot survey. The researchers felt that the subject of pressure sores crossed all professional and organizational boundaries and hence included doctors, nurses and therapists in the survey. On the medical side the questionnaire was circulated to all registrars, senior house officers and house officers. The consultants were omitted because some were working on a pressure sore policy. All clinical nurse managers,

Table 9.2 Advice

- 4% seek advice from nursing staff
- 4% from nursing and medical staff
- 5% from all staff (including therapists)
- 6% from medical staff
- 3% from nursing and therapy staff
- 3% did not seek advice
- 1.5% seek advice from all sources

ward sisters and charge nurses as well as all heads of the therapy services and senior 1 and senior 11 occupational and physiotherapists were included.

A total of 324 questionnaires were sent out with a 41% response rate (29% of medical staff, 45% of nursing staff, 79% of OT staff and 33% of physiotherapists). The results indicated that a majority of nurses and therapists routinely assessed patients regarding pressure sore risk, while very few junior doctors did so. Approximately half the responding nursing staff used some form of assessment scale or scoring system for pressure sores (e.g. Norton, Waterlow); hardly any junior doctors or therapy staff did so. The majority of nurses and about half the responding therapists and doctors were aware of a standard classification for pressure sores.

Sixty two percent of the responders were unaware of any hospital/ward pressure care policy. When it came to seeking advice from other staff members when an inpatient developed a pressure sore, the results can be seen in Table 9.2.

Other groups from whom advice was sought included pharmacists, patient, plastic surgery department, disablement service centres, district nurses, rehabilitation engineers, community team, Wound Care Association, pressure sore advisor, seating clinic, chiropodist and medical representatives. The feedback on the total cost of inpatient treatment of pressure sores varied from less than £100 in 3% of responders to between £1000 and £10 000 as regards the total treatment costs in 39%.

The authors felt that a surprisingly large number of responders (97%) were aware of the specialized equipment available for pressure management; 78% were keen or felt a need to attend courses/lectures demonstrating this equipment. Some of the comments reproduced in the article are illuminating.

The importance of pressure sores, I feel, is recognized by medical staff, yet their identification and expertise in management is very much thought to be with the field of nursing.

The fact that pressure sores arise in the first place is a failure of nursing staff recognition of at-risk patients and inadequate prophylaxis. Ward staff shortages do not help this situation.

Often it is not a lack of knowledge that causes pressure sores but a lack of resources.

The authors confirmed that the medical staff were poor responders to the questionnaire as the subject of pressure sores is not considered a priority issue. In addition medical staff rarely routinely assessed patients with regard to pressure sore risk and, with therapy staff, were unaware of any assessment protocols to help. There was an overall lack of awareness of the true costs of pressure sores.

To try and combat the medical nihilism that prevents adequate undergraduate teaching on chronic wounds, some medical schools/ colleges have revolutionized the undergraduate teaching curriculum.

Medical students at the London Hospital Medical College spend most of their clinical attachments at the constituent hospitals of the Royal London Hospital (Whitechapel, Mile End and St Clements). The Department of Health Care of the Elderly (DHCE) has always incorporated a core lecture concerning chronic wounds and pressure sores in particular within its two-week teaching and clinical attachment block. In 1992 the whole medical undergraduate curriculum was reviewed and modified. Previously the DHCE received its students in two-week rotations in their final year. The new curriculum, through much planning and mutual consent, resulted in the creation of an eight-week block in the students' first clinical year consisting of Clinical Epidemiology, General Practice and Health Care of the Elderly.

The course organizers are endeavouring to produce a 'seamless' approach to these three subjects. The teaching objectives are geared to demonstrate the way in which the same relevant themes are found in each of the separate entities. Professional barriers are notoriously hard to break down yet this course is having some success.

The medical students begin their eight weeks with an introduction to the three components of the block and a description of how relevant they are to each other. Within the total time there are three phases recognizable, with Clinical Epidemiology moving into Health Care of the Elderly and then onto General Practice. Initially the key word was integration. In order to try and achieve this the concept of a course assignment was developed. This is a form of project that the students have to develop and present both as an oral report to their peers and as a written set of notes (for their colleagues not doing the same assignment). The themes of the assignments are chosen because of their suitability to demonstrate an integrated approach. The students are given a framework of notes on the assignment chosen and in week 1 of the course meet their assignment tutors. There is a lead or primary tutor for each topic but also secondary tutors so that expertise is available from the three core subjects.

One of the assignments is Chronic Wounds. The lead tutor is a consultant in care of the elderly and the secondary tutors include the clinical nurse specialist in tissue viability and a general practice nurse with expertise in chronic wounds. Epidemiological and statistical advice is available. The tutor's role is to enthuse the students about the subject and introduce them to the framework notes. They meet the students regularly throughout the eight weeks and help them prepare for the final presentation. However, the students are encouraged to use self-directed learning (SDL) techniques and be innovative in both what they choose to concentrate on within the framework and how they present the material. The student notes given to all are meant to fill in the knowledge base gaps for the other students. Themes within the assignment include disease management (DM), health promotion (HP) and service management (SM). The framework notes given to the Chronic Wound assignment students (including references) are reproduced below.

London Hospital Medical College Phase 111 Curriculum

Clinical Epidemiology/General Practice/Department of Health Care of the Elderly Assignments

CHRONIC WOUNDS

Chronic wounds being defined for the purposes of the assignment as leg ulcers (all types), pressure sores and other non-healing wounds. At the start of the assignment students will need to have or to gain knowledge of the common clinical forms and pathological causes of chronic wounds. The aim should be that this is broadly achieved before the start of the DHCE attachment (i.e. in the introductory session and in the early section of DHCE/applied epidemiology). This knowledge will continue to expand during the following six weeks.

Part of the assignment requires each student to write up two case studies of chronic wounds. The subjects for these will be found in the DHCE and General Practice. The ten or so case studies so produced will more than cover the common clinical forms (venous leg ulcers, arterial leg ulcers, diabetic leg ulcers, superficial and deep pressure sores and other non-healing wounds).

The order of the sections below is significant. Groups ought to achieve sections 1 to 6. Sections 7 and 8 are more optional and might be replaced by other subprojects.

Medical history of chronic wounds

In what ways may the historic figures in wound care have influenced modern practice?

References

Bennett, G.C.J. (1992) Pressure sores, in *Textbook of Geriatric Medicine and Gerontology* 4th edn, (eds J.C. Brocklehurst, R.C. Tallis and H.M. Fillit), Churchill Livingstone, Edinburgh.

Daniel, R.K. (1979) Pressure sores – a reappraisal. *Ann Plastic Surg*, **1**, 53–63.

Charcot, J.M. (1877) *Lectures on the Diseases of the Nervous System. Delivered at La Saltpetriere* (trans. G. Sigerson), New Sydenham Society, London.

Incidence and prevalence

What is known about the hospital and community incidence and prevalence of leg ulcers and pressure sores?

References

Bennett, G.C.J. (1992) Pressure sores, in *Textbook of Geriatric Medicine and Gerontology*, 4th edn, (eds J.C. Brocklehurst, R.C. Tallis and H.M. Fillit), Churchill Livingstone, Edinburgh.

Bennett, G.C.J. and Ebrahim, S. (1992) *Essentials of Health Care of the Elderly*, Edward Arnold, London.

Aetiology

What are the aetiological factors? Have they changed over time (with reference to Medical History of Chronic Wounds)?

References

Bennett, G.C.J. (1992) Pressure sores, in *Textbook of Geriatric Medicine and Gerontology*, 4th edn, (eds J.C. Brocklehurst, R.C. Tallis and H.M. Fillit), Churchill Livingstone, Edinburgh.

Bader, D. (1991) *Pressure Sores: Science and Practice*, Macmillan, Basingstoke.

Prevention

What can individuals, hospitals, general practitioners and government do to reduce the incidence and recurrence rate of chronic wounds?

This could involve consideration of screening, patient education, professional education, risk assessment scales, cost, cost–benefit ratios, litigation, defensive medicine.

References

Bliss, M. Pressure sores. Textbok of Geriatric Medicine and Gerontology. 4th Edition. Ed. Brocklehurst 1992.
Bennett, G.C.J. and Ebrahim, S. Essentials of Health Care of the Elderly. Pressure Sores. Edward Arnold 1992.

Management of chronic wounds

Aetiology influencing management, wound assessment, moist wound healing, bandages, dressings, drugs, mechanical aids, cost.

References

Royal London NHS Trust Wound Care Formulary (and ask clinical nurse specialist on tissue viability).

Health service planning

Devise the most cost effective and efficient local service delivery for people with leg ulcers and pressure sores.

References

Published works by C. Moffat re Riverside Health Authority/Charing Cross leg ulcer project.
Published works by K. Harding, Director Wound Healing Research Unit, University Hospital of Wales, Cardiff.

Cutting edge: treatment and research techniques

What is the role of cultured skin grafts, growth factors and hyperbaric oxygen in the treatment of chronic wounds? Discuss the value of transcutaneous oxygen and carbon dioxide monitoring, laser Doppler and ultrasound as research techniques.

> **Medical ethics and legal issues**
>
> Discuss what should happen if a patient develops a pressure sore in hospital. How can one determine failure of care? What is the redress (including legal?). Many chronic wounds are present in people who are not mentally competent; should research treatments (ranging from new dressings to the use of growth factors) be permitted?

The importance of chronic wounds in the medical undergraduate curriculum within the Department of Health Care of the Elderly is further reinforced by a lecture on chronic wounds, especially pressure sores, and, from January 1994, a day's experience on the newly opened wound care unit. This exciting venture between the Departments of Clinical Dermatology and Health Care of the Elderly has resulted in a four-bed inpatient facility for the assessment and treatment of chronic wounds, particularly in the older client. In addition, there is an outpatient clinic for difficult or slow to heal wounds and joint inpatient rounds with a dermatologist and a clinician in care of the elderly. Thus students will have an insight into the range of wound care issues, from basic wounds to complex multidisciplinary problems.

UNDERGRADUATE TEXTBOOKS

There is a dearth of educational material concerning chronic wounds aimed at the undergraduate (or indeed the postgraduate) medical student. In 1992, however, the Centre for Medical Education based at the University of Dundee, Scotland, produced *The Wound Programme*. This softback, beautifully illustrated and produced book has an excellent production team including Keith Harding, Director of the Wound Healing Research Unit, University of Wales College of Medicine, Peta Dunkley, Lecturer in Surgery and Associate Director of the Surgical Skills unit, University of Dundee, and Ronald M. Harden, Professor of Medical Education, University of Dundee.

It does not aim to be a conventional comprehensive textbook on wound care. Instead it aims to direct the student to try and understand the concept of wound healing using clinical case examples of wound injury from different causes. *The Wound Programme* has five components:

Part A The Reader's Guide

This consists of information about the programme and how to use it.

Part B Patient Management Challenges

This provides the student with a clinically based example (plus photograph) of a type of wound. Information about that patient's problem is presented with a series of questions divided into subgroups:

- structure and function of skin;
- pathology and microbiology;
- causes, appearances and management;
- management in the community;
- questions for experienced practitioners.

The student can then compare their management decision with that of an expert in the field.

Part C What You Need to Know about Wounds

This section details the important facts that students will need to apply when managing patients with wounds. The information is presented in the context of a unique Wound Organizer. It emphasizes the six aspects which must be considered every time a patient with a wound is assessed and managed:

1. Site
2. Stage
3. Cause
4. Form
5. Environment and carer
6. Health care system.

These aspects are expanded upon and their inter-relationships described. The Wound Organizer gives the student:

- a framework for learning;
- a format for the content material;
- an Organizer to enable the student to assess and manage patients with wounds.

Part D Glossary

This is an explanation of the terminology used in the book.

Part E   Consensus Statement

This reproduces a document from the International Committee on Wound Management, an international group of experts, reviewing general principles for the management of patients with wounds.

Further information about the availability of *The Wound Programme* for use with medical undergraduate teaching can be obtained from the Centre for Medical Education, University of Dundee, Scotland.

Some medical schools/colleges in England, Scotland and Wales provide their medical students with a sound knowledge base concerning chronic wounds and wound healing. Most do not, leaving those graduates the daunting task of learning 'on the job'. This is unsatisfactory for both doctor as well as patient. Both deserve better.

NURSE EDUCATION

The demands upon nurses and the demands made by nurses are constantly changing in an endeavour to keep pace with the goals of the organization.

Adaptability and flexibility [3] are essential prerequisites for the competent practitioner. However, whatever constitutes competence today, we can be sure its meaning will have changed by tomorrow, therefore the foundation for future professional competence seems to be the capacity to learn how to learn [4]. There are many difficulties facing a profession that continues to educate itself largely by a process of osmosis [5–7] and which has drawn heavily on the medical model as the foundation for its professional education and development given that the use of such models inhibits or detracts from the development of skills and knowledge required as a basis for individual patient care [8] and application of critical thinking skills.

The need for nurses to extend their role has been postulated by many medical and nursing practitioners and a framework has been provided by the UKCC [9]. However, although some medical staff appear to want intelligent observers capable of conducting highly technical procedures, some still expect the nurse to be a person who primarily follows instructions [10] which, in issues related to wound management, can result in friction between medical and nursing practitioners.

Education has several well established and important functions. These include the presentation and transmission of knowledge (the teaching and learning function), the extension of knowledge (the research function) and the training in advanced skills needed by society [11].

The function of nurse education is to prepare and develop learners to act as competent professional practitioners. The Nurses, Midwives and Health Visitors Act [12] introduced considerable debate within the profession about how best to educate and train nurses to meet the changing demands of society and the goals of the health care service. This debate intensified from the summer of 1984, when the UKCC established a project to determine the education and training required for nursing in relation to the projected health care needs in the 1990s and beyond. This culminated in the publication of the report *Project 2000 – A New Preparation for Practice* [13] laying the foundation for nursing courses to be properly recognized by academic institutions. The project team stated that to survive in a turbulent environment and at a time when cost saving and reallocation of resources are on the agenda, nurses must be prepared to accept challenges to their practice and to evaluate and review their performance [14].

By 1985 impatience at the UKCC delay in publishing concrete proposals led to the Royal College of Nursing Commission on Nurse Education and the English National Board Consultation Paper [15] on professional education and training courses. Both had considerable influence on the recommendations finally made to government.

The suggestion that education exists to help individuals to grow and develop their potential as opposed to helping to shape and mould them to suit the ideas and ideals of teachers is not an entirely new concept; such claims were made by Socrates [16]. The effectiveness of traditional teaching styles has been questioned and challenged [17–19] due to their inability to encourage creativity or critical and analytic thinking skills, whereas the main aims of progressive education include assisting the recipient to deal with situations more realistically, discussing subjective and objective perspectives, encouraging critical and analytic thinking, promoting active learning and the transference of learning from one situation to another [20].

The philosophical ethics of many nurse education programmes are based on a humanistic perspective of personal growth and development, self-direction and self and peer review using principles drawn from the theory of andragogy postulated by Knowles [21] and based on four fundamental functions:

1. concept of the learner;
2. role of learner's experience;
3. readiness to learn;
4. orientation to learning.

Adults tend to have a deep psychological need to be generally self-directing and each experience provides an increasingly rich source of learning which furthers personal growth and development [21].

For a person to cope more effectively with real life problems or situations they experience a need and readiness to learn at certain times in their lives. Education may therefore be viewed as the process of developing increased competence through the facilitation of the learner's interaction with their environment, a process which requires a change in the curriculum and the role of the nurse teacher.

Over the years there has been increasing emphasis on the importance of evaluation in the health care service, including educational and training programmes, which provides a systematic examination of a whole course in order to bring about improvements and development in the course programme [22].

The actual nature and function of evaluation has changed over the years to meet the programme demands, with certain values or qualities being identified as worthwhile to the development of an educational programme and becoming the criteria against which all aspects of that programme are judged. As society's views on what is valuable change, so do aspects of the educational programme. Therefore the criteria by which we judge anything reflects the prevailing values of the times, which in disciplines allied to science depend to some extent on the current state of knowledge [23].

In March 1994, the UKCC issued a Position Statement on policy and implementation for the future of professional practice – the Councils' standards for education and practice following registration [30]. These standards include three major sets of requirements:

1. standards for a period of support for newly registered practitioners, under the guidance of a preceptor;
2. standards for maintaining an effective registration;
3. standards for postregistration education.

The standards relating to maintaining an effective registration and to postregistration education are statutory requirements. The former applies to all practitioners requiring an effective registration with the Council. The latter applies to those seeking a specialist qualification in nursing or specialist community health care nursing.

Advanced nursing practice is concerned with adjusting the boundaries for the development of future practice, pioneering and developing new roles responsive to clinical practice, research and education to enrich professional practice as a whole. The continuing development of the professional [29] is in the interests of patients, clients and the health service.

There are an increasing number of clinical nurse specialists in tissue viability and wound care but as yet no recognized specialist qualification for the practitioners who hold these posts. The first ENB course on leg ulcers was developed at Charing Cross; more recently, the Institute of Health and Community Services, University of Bournemouth, has produced a range of open, mixed mode and taught courses, up to and including a Masters level, to meet the differing needs of nurses and other health care professions on these important subject areas. Many nurses rely on keeping up to date by reading professional journals and attending ad hoc study days. Open learning and taught courses are now being developed to meet the educational needs of the evolving group of specialist nurses.

Commercial sponsorship and innovation have greatly contributed to the development and application of knowledge. The provision of study days, purchase of course places, production and provision of educational material and the support of advisory services are among the many activities offered by commercial companies.

REGULATION OF THE PROFESSION

Nursing, midwifery and health visiting in the United Kingdom have been regulated by the United Kingdom Central Council (UKCC) following its inception as part of the Nurses, Midwives and Health Visitors Act 1979. Section $2^{(1)}$ of the Act states that the principal functions of the Central Council shall be to establish and improve standards of training and professional conduct [12].

The Code of Professional Conduct for the Nurse, Midwife and Health Visitor is the Council's definitive advice on professional conduct to its practitioners [25] to ensure that a minimum safe standard of care is provided at all times, in such a manner as to justify public trust and confidence, uphold and enhance the good standing and reputation of the professional, to serve the interests of society and above all, to safeguard the interests of individual patients and clients [25] who often, when they are at their most dependent and vulnerable, have no option but to place themselves in the care of people who are professionally qualified to respond to their needs [26]. The independence and impartiality of the profession are seen as important characteristics by the public; hence it is important, during the current attempts to make the National Health Service more like a business, to ensure professional behaviour is not unwillingly altered.

The Code also provides the backcloth against which any alleged misconduct on the part of the nurse will be judged [24].

Accountability for one's actions is an integral part of professional practice. It is an accepted fact that the practitioner will have to make judgements in a wide variety of situations and circumstances and be answerable for those judgements. The Code of Conduct does not seek to state all the circumstances in which accountability has to be exercised, but to state important principles. The UKCC recognizes that in many situations in which practitioners practise there may be a tension between maintenance of standards and the availability or use of resources, but it expects its practitioners to seek remedies in those situations where factors in the environment obstruct the achievement of high standards. To start from a compromise position and silently to tolerate poor standards is to act in a manner contrary to the interests of patients or clients and thus renege on personal and professional accountability. Some practitioners may object to participation in certain forms of treatment that are prescribed, including the use of wound dressings. If the practitioner believes (from knowledge, published research evidence or from previous experience) that the prescribed substance (topical solution or wound dressing) may be harmful, or even more so where it is evident that it is actively harmful, they should make a record of the condition of the wound or site (where appropriate including a photographic record) and ask the prescribing medical practitioner to attend. If the prescription stands after medical examination, the practitioner, having chosen either to respond to the prescription or not, should make a detailed record of the reasons for their expressed concern and subsequent action [24]. The UKCC believe that the spirit of collaboration, cooperation and mutual respect for the contribution of other members of the multidisciplinary team should make such actions an exception rather than a rule.

THE CONCEPT OF NURSING/MEDICAL NEGLIGENCE

In order to establish negligence in a civil action for damages the plaintiff (the patient) or his representative must show that the investigation, diagnosis and/or treatment of the plaintiff's condition fell below the standard of reasonably competent practitioners in their respective fields [27].

The test for assessing criticism of the investigation, diagnosis or treatment is whether the allegations can be justified on the 'balance of probability', more likely than not, rather than the more rigorous standard of proof 'beyond reasonable doubt' amounting to the certainty required in criminal cases.

The burden of proof in cases of negligence clearly rests with the plaintiff or his representative who must demonstrate to the court that on the balance of probabilities, the practitioner (and/or their employer who may be held vicariously liable) was under a legal duty of care, that there was a breach of the appropriate standard of care and that the plaintiff suffered harm or damage as a result of that breach [28].

Nursing negligence in relation to tissue viability and wound care can arise because of professional adherence to tradition where custom and practice prevail rather than the application of relevant research based findings as the basis of decision making. Negligence may also arise out of a failure to act. The nurse has a responsibility to draw attention to any situation which may be harmful to the patient, hence advocacy is an essential feature in the exercising of accountability and lack of professional knowledge, skill or awareness of a situation is not a defence. Practitioners must therefore possess a sound knowledge and skill base to remain competent.

It is a defence to an allegation of professional negligence for a defendant to prove that a substantial body of reputable practitioners in the field would have carried out the investigation or treatment in the same way as those against whom allegations are made, even if the decision behind the investigation or treatment is found to have been mistaken. It is advised for both plaintiff and defendant to refer to at least one contemporary authoritative publication for each criticism or defence.

Most nurses are fully aware of the responsibilities associated with their evolving role in this litigious society, yet they frequently fail to provide clear and concise nursing records [29].

Adopting a holistic approach to patient assessment and care combined with accurate record keeping will assist practitioners to view their role with greater satisfaction and be more confident about making professional judgements or justifying the level of intervention for their patients.

REFERENCES

1. Bennett, G. (1992) Undergraduate teaching on chronic wound care. *Lancet*, **339**, 249–50.
2. Kulkarni, J. and Philbin, M. (1993) Pressure sore awareness in a university teaching hospital. *J Tissue Viability*, **3**(3), 77–9.
3. Georgopoulous, B.S. and Mann, F.C. (1972) The hospital as an organisation, in *Patients, Physicians and Illness*, (ed. J.E. Gartly), The Free Press, New York.
4. Argyn, C. and Schon, D.A. (1974) *Theory in Practice. Increasing Professional Effectiveness*, Jossey-Bass, San Francisco.
5. Auld, M. (1979) Nursing in a changing society. *J Adv Nursing*, **4**, 287–98.
6. Hunter, T.D. (1971) New ways in health care management. *Br Hosp Soc Service Rev*, **81**(4237), 1319–20.

7. Roper, N. (1976) *Clinical Experience in Nurse Education*, Monograph Number 5, Dept of Nursing Studies, University of Edinburgh.
8. Akinsanya, J. and Hayward, J. (1980). The biological sciences in nurse education. *Nursing Times*, **76**(11), 427–32.
9. UKCC (1994) Scope of Professional Practice, UKCC, London.
10. Anderson, E.R. (1973). *The Role of the Nurse*, Royal College of Nursing, London.
11. Cox, G. (1982) The seeds of time – or the future of nurse education. *Nurse Educ Today*, **2**(1), 4–10.
12. Department of Health and Social Security (1979) *The Nurses, Midwives and Health Visitors Act*, HMSO, London.
13. United Kingdom Central Council (1986) *Project 2000 – A New Preparation for Practice*, UKCC, London.
14. UKCC (1987) *Project 2000 –The Final Proposal*, Project Paper 9. UKCC, London.
15. English National Board (1985) *Professional Education and Training Courses*, Consultation Paper, ENB, London.
16. Moody, M. (1989) Evaluation of a pilot sister development scheme. Unpublished MPhil thesis, Southampton University.
17. Bloom, B., Englehart, M., Furst, E. *et al.* (1974) *Taxonomy of Educational Objectives. Handbook 1 Cognitive Domain.* Longman, London.
18. Hellinworth, B. (1979) Teaching the nursing process: a challenge for nurse teachers. *Nursing Times*, **75**(30), 1263.
19. Darwin, J. (1980) Obedience is not enough. *Nursing Mirror*, **146**(2), 32–5.
20. Cooper, S.E. (1981) Methods of teaching revisited – care method. *J Cont Educ Nursing*, **12**(5), 32–6.
21. Knowles, M. (1980) *Modern Practice of Adult Education*, revised edn, Prentice-Hall, Cambridge, Mass.
22. Joint Board of Clinical Studies (1979) *Course Evaluation Package*, Occasional Publication , JBCS, London.
23. Allen, H.O. (1982) *The Ward Sister: Role and Preparation*, Ballière Tindall, London.
24. UKCC (1989) *Exercising Accountability*, a UKCC Advisory Document, UKCC London.
25. UKCC (1992) *Code of Professional Conduct for the Nurse, Midwife and Health Visitor*, 3rd edn, UKCC, London.
26. Pyne, R. (1993) Accountability in wound care (1). The UKCC Directive. *Wound Man*, **3**(1), 5–6.
27. Young, A.P. (1991) *Law and Professional Conduct in Nursing*, Scutari Press, London.
28. Moore, D. (1992) *Wound Management – an Ethicolegal Perspective*, Institute of Health and Community Services, University of Bournemouth.
29. Moody, M. (1993) Accountability in wound care (2). A practical approach. *Wound Man*, **3**(1), 6–7.
30. UKCC (1994) *The Future of Professional Practice – The Council's Standard for Education and Practice Following Registration*, Position Statement on Policy and Implementation, UKCC, London.

FURTHER READING

Baker, J. (1988) *What next? Postbasic Opportunities for Nurses*, Macmillan Education, Basingstoke.

Butterworth, T. and Faugier, J. (eds) (1992) *Clinical Supervision and Mentorship in Nursing*, Chapman & Hall, London.

Dimond, B. (1990) *Legal Aspects of Nursing*, Prentice-Hall, London.

Robinson, J., Gray, A. and Elkan, R. (eds) (1992) *Policy Issues in Nursing*, Open University, Milton Keynes.

Index

Page numbers appearing in **bold** refer to figures and page numbers appearing in *italic* refer to tables.